AF342169

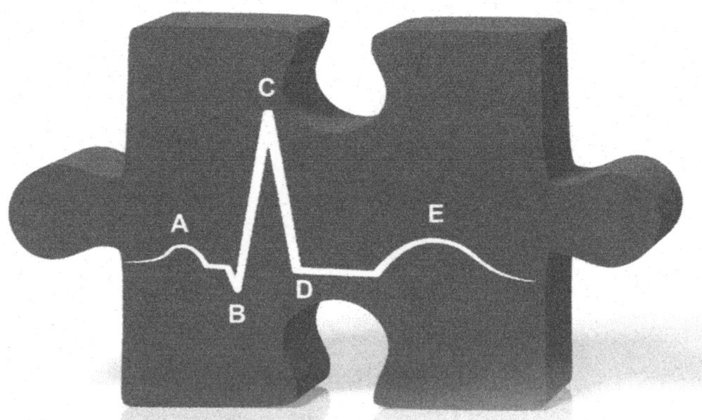

PUZZLES
IN RESUSCITATING MCQs EXAM

FOR MEDICAL STUDENTS
AND SURGICAL RESIDENTS

(1ST Edition)

DISCLAIMERS

The author has made all the effort to check the copyright of all borrowed information. If he overlooked any, he would make the appropriate arrangement at the first **opportunity**.

The author has taken all the care to check that the information presented is accurate and up to the current practice. However, the author cannot be held responsible for any errors or consequences from the application of the information. Practitioners are fully responsible for the application of the provided information in a particular situation.

TABLE OF CONTENTS

PUZZLE I

PREREADING MCQ EXAM..**3**

PUZZLE II

PRE-EXAM STRATEGY..**7**

PUZZLE III

INTRA-EXAM STRATEGY...**17**

PUZZLE IV

POST-EXAM STRATEGY **25**

PUZZLE V

RECOVERY STRATEGY **27**

PREFACE

Saving your multiple-choice question (MCQ) exam needs knowledge and skills. You have seen colleagues who are not bothered with the exam and they do not study for it, but when you look at their results, you get shocked. You start asking yourself, "How come they have a good score even when they did not study?" There are two possibilities. First, they pretend that they do not study (sick people). Second, they have strategies in dealing with the exam (lucky people). Advanced MCQ Life Support (AMLS) will make you one of those geeks. It will show you how to deal with MCQ exam like a patient and teach you how to approach the exam when the situation is stable and when you start losing control (examic shock: exam-induced shock). It is fun to read and you can finish it before you go to bed like bedtime story. You will get addicted to this book and will keep reading it again and again until you fall asleep. This mini book will improve your score in the MCQ exam especially when your knowledge and experience fail **you**.

ACKNOWLEDGMENT

There are a few extraordinary people who contributed to this book in different ways. My parents provided me with all the support, guidance, and love to be successful and to be able to write this book. Without them, after God's will, I would have not made it this far. My siblings were there every time I needed to vent out my stress. Marring my wife Sawsan was the beginning of endless success. She is always there when I need her. She contributed to this with her love, patience, and imagination. I am thankful to my kids for keeping the smile on my face and for nourishing my life with love and happiness. Finally, I would like to thank my geek colleagues who made me think that there is more than just knowledge to SAVE YOUR MCQ **EXAM!**

PUZZLE I
PREREADING MCQ EXAM

BEFORE YOU START READING THIS BOOK

You must go through the following ten MCQs as prereading assessment. Try to answer them in the best way you think will make you score the highest. In a separate paper, make a table with four columns. First column is for the question number; second column, for you prereading answer; third column, leave it for you post-reading answers; and the fourth column is used to comment on the result of your pre – and post-reading questions (i.e. Did your score improve? Did your score remain the same or got worse after your finished reading this book? What type of strategy have you used to answer it?). These questions are NOT medical because I would like to reduce the chance that you will use your knowledge to answer **them**.

PREREADING 10 MCQS

1. What is the capital of Mexico?

    A. Rio de Janeiro

    B. Veracruz

    C. Ciudad de México

    D. Tabasco City

    E. Salvador

2. Sentinelese is a ward used to describe a

    A. Ancient animal

    B. Tribe

    C. Isolated island

    D. Irish family existed in the past

    E. Organized community in South America

3. Which of the following countries lie on the Equator?

    A. Panama

    B. India

    C. Democratic Republic of the Congo

    D. United Arab of Emirates

    E. Malaysia

4. What would be the most common cause of malpractice suits against physicians?

    A. Failure to diagnose is not uncommon

    B. Incorrect surgery

    C. Errors in medication administration

    D. Poor documentation

    E. Failure to treat

5. What is correct about Paris Saint Germain football club?

    A. Always win the cup

    B. Red–Blue uniform

    C. Never disappoint their fans

    D. Red–Black uniform

    E. Originally from Monte Carlo

6. Which of the following own an island in the Caribbean?

    A. France

    B. United Kingdom

    C. United States of America

    D. All of the above

    E. None of the above

7. Which are the main gases present in the Sun?

    A. Hydrogen and Argon

    B. Oxygen and Carbon dioxide

    C. Nitrogen and Carbon monoxide

    D. Hydrogen and Helium

    E. Nitrogen oxide

8. According to the Occupational Safety and Health Administration (OSHA), informational safety sheets must be present in art rooms that contain which of the following safety risks?

    A. Sharp objects

    B. Loud noises

    C. Heat-producing machinery

    D. Visual hazard

    E. Hazardous and risky chemicals

9. Which of the following are components of Central Processing Unit (CPU) in your computer?

A. Mouse and monitor
B. Control unit and USP outlets
C. Arithmetic logic unit and control unit
D. Keyboard and mouse
E. Integrated circuits

10. Which of the following country has/have pyramids?

A. Sudan
B. Mexico
C. Italy
D. Both A and B
E. Both B and C
F. All A, B, and C

PUZZLE II
PRE-EXAM STRATEGY

INTRODUCTION

Fear, sweating, palpitation, cold hands, tremor, and about to lose consciousness, all are symptoms of shock. This is what we call it examic (examination-induced) shock. I am sure that you have faced this feeling many times in your life. Because you are reading this book, it means that you try to know how to save your MCQ examination. As you know, when a patient arrests, you have to perform cardiopulmonary resuscitation (CPR) to bring your patient back by following the guidelines of Advanced Cardiac Life Support (ACLS®). For unstable MCQ exam, you must follow Advanced MCQ Life Support (AMLS).

To save it, you should know it!

Knowing your patient is essential for you to know it. You should know the anatomy, physiology (function of MCQ exam), and pathology (what cam goes wrong with the exam) of the MCQ **exam.**

Multiple (M): means that you have more than one sentence

Choice (C): means that you have to select from a list of choices

Questions (Q): set of question or exercises evaluating skill or knowledge

Therefore, MCQ is a type of exam that depends on selecting the answer that you think it is RIGHT!

HISTORY

The main tool that is used to assess the knowledge of the students for hundreds of years is through exams. The number of students is increasing every day, and the need for a rapid and effective evaluation initiated the utilization of the MCQ as a quantitative and qualitative tool. MCQs have a long history, which was started by E. Thorndike, the educational psychologist, who developed an early multiple-choice test. In 1914, Frederick J. Kelly, Dean of the College of Education at the University of Kansas, introduced the multiple-choice test. The Army Alpha performed the first multiple-choice, large-scale assessment. It was used to assess the intelligence of the World War I military **recruits**.

ETIOLOGY

Why MCQ test existed and why it became the most popular method of assessment when compared to other types of tests? You have to know that MCQ is the most popular type used worldwide, even though it is not the easiest. There are plenty of reasons that make them so beloved by the examiners and preferred by **students**:

- It requires much less time than essay exam, where you have to prove your point by listing points or explanations.
- Multiple-choice tests are strong and fair predictors of overall student performance (objective) unlike other forms of evaluations, as written and essay exam, in-class participation, case exams, assignments, and presentation, which could be very subjective.
- One doesn't need to spend a lot of time in studying and memorizing every word. Test takers need just to understand the whole idea and the general concepts of the subject.
- It is clear and easy for students to go through and ideal for examiner to mark it because a software will do it for them.
- Bad hand-writers do not face an issue.

CLASSIFICATION (see Figure 1)

Unfortunately, exam is the dark side of medical student's life, and the student has to go through countless tests. Therefore, you need to find out what types of exams you might encounter and at what **stage**:

1 – Collage Acceptance Exams

All over the world, high school graduates undergo a college entrance exam, which is used to help in selecting specific number of students to get accepted into the collage. Medical schools are using a standardized entrance test to select the top students among the applicants due to the limited seats available.

2 – Medical School Exams

I. Academic years: include exams in basic science such as Anatomy, Biochemistry, and Physiology.

II. Clinical years: include exams in Internal Medicine, General Surgery, Pediatric, Obstetrics and Gynecology, and other branches.

3 – Licensing Exams

Exams that enable you to get acceptance in board residency program:

I. United States Medical Licensing Examination (USMLE)

    a. USMLE Step 1: Basic science Examination

    b. USMLE Step 2: Clinical knowledge and clinical skills

    c. USMLE Step 3: Final assessment of physicians assuming independent responsibility for delivering general medical care

II. Medical Council of Canada Evaluating Examination (MCCEE): tests clinical knowledge

III. Professional and Linguistic Assessments Board (PLAB)

IV. The PLAB test is the main route by which International Medical Graduates (IMG) demonstrate that they have the necessary skills and knowledge to practice medicine in the United Kingdom

V. Saudi Medical License Examination (SMLE)

a. Saudi Licensing Exam (SMLE) for medical specialty or general practice licensing

b. It is essential to allow you to work in Saudi Arabia and to get accepted in Saudi residency programs

4 – Residency Program Exams

I. Annual exams: to assess the progress of the resident

II. Qualifying exam: to allow the student to enter the final exam

III. Certifying exam: specialty-specific final exam

5 – Special Nonmedical Exams

It includes all the exams, such as the English Language Exams, that are needed in order to get accepted in certain programs in different **countries**:

I. *Test of English as a Foreign Language* (TOFEL): an English-language test. More than 8,500 colleges, universities, and agencies in more than 130 countries, including Australia, Canada, UK, and the USA, recognize this exam

II. *International English Language Testing System* (IELTS): an English-language test. More than 7,000 institutions in 135 countries recognize this exam

Exam Classification
Collage acceptance exams
Medical school exams
Licensing exams
Residency program exams
Special non-medical exams
Academic exams
Clinical exams
USMLE
MCCEE
PLAP
SMLE
Others
English language
Annual exams
Qualifiying exam
Certifyig exam

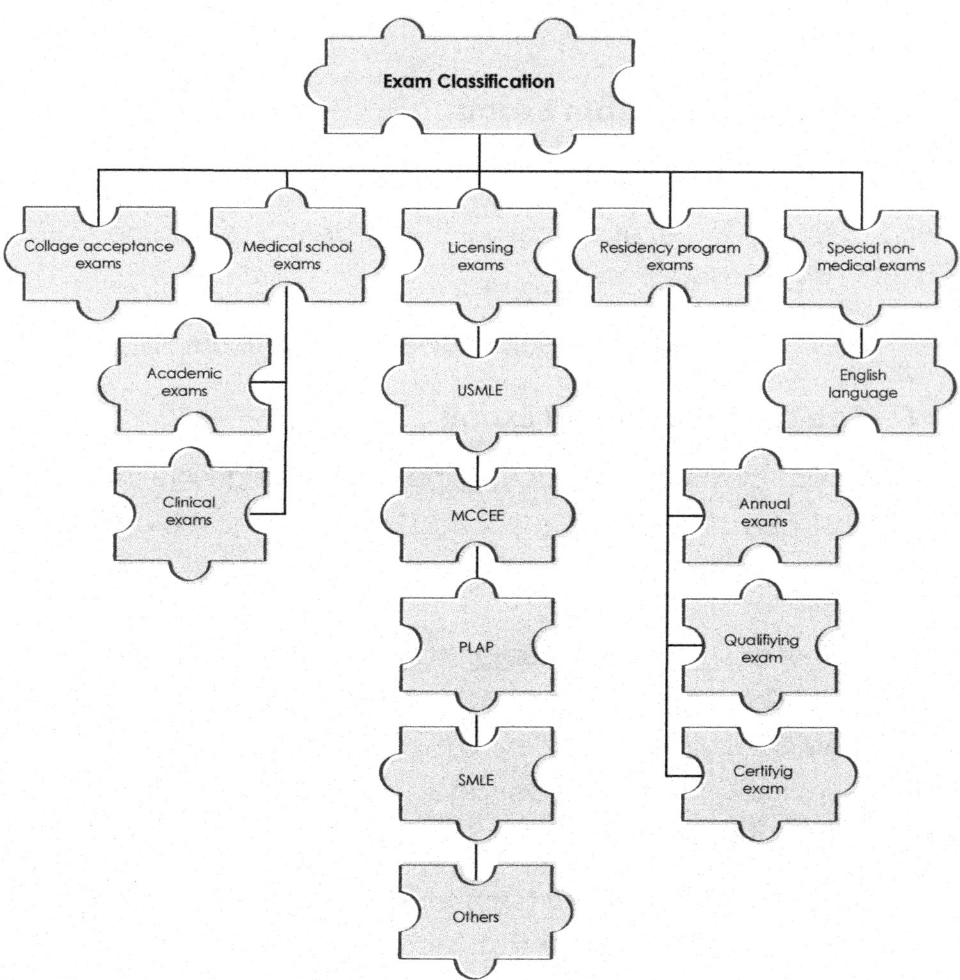

Figure 1

TYPES OF MCQ EXAMS

"What does MCQ exam test mean you for?" This is a very common question each student would like to answer. There are two types of MCQ exam based on the skill that is **testing**:

- Recognition and Recall: Depends purely on your ability to memorize the information. It tests the lowest level of student's cognitive function because it depends on the recall skills only.
- Analytic and Reasoning: Depends less on memorization but more on understanding and analyzing the information. It tests a higher level of cognitive function.

ANATOMY OF MCQ (see Figure **2**)

Take a close look at the anatomy of your enemy and try to analyze it. The body of the MCQ consists of the following:

- The question itself, which is called the "Stem"
- The best correct answer, which is called the "Key Answer"
- The less correct or incorrect answers, which are called the "Distracters"

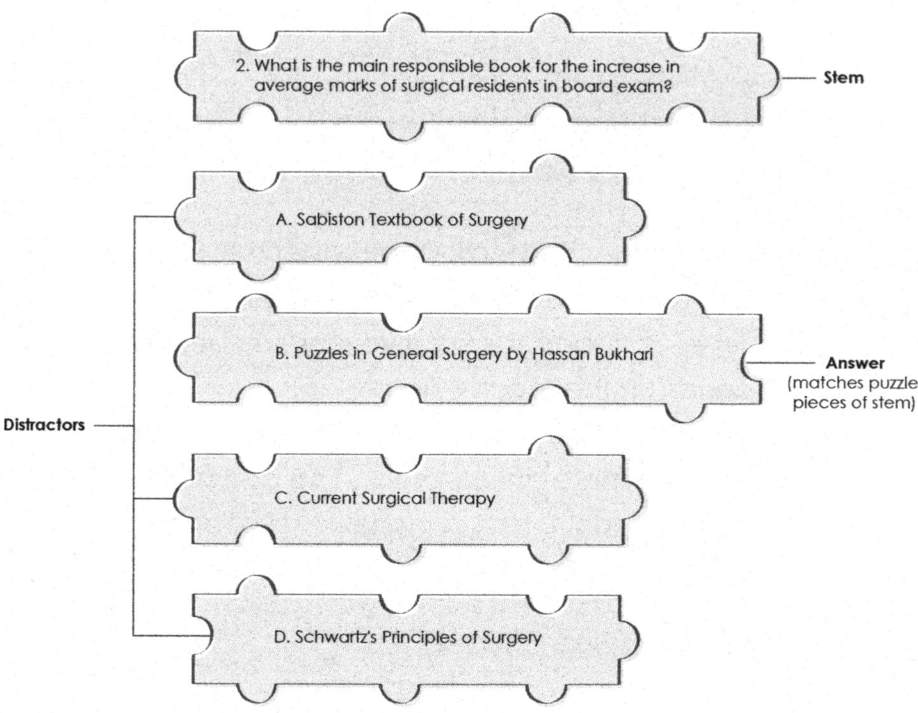

Figure 2

MANAGEMENT

There are few critical management approaches to be taken into consideration before the day of exam. Superb preparation, relaxation, and avoiding any unnecessary stressful (have enough stress) situations are the **key**.

Superb Preparation

- Focus well on what your instructor/lecture emphasized.
- Make your own notes, lists, tables, and algorithms.

- Challenge your colleagues daily with difficult MCQs (brainstorming) to embarrass them intentionally so they will come next day with more difficult MCQs for revenge!! (This will benefit you and your colleagues in the long run.)
- Start preparing for your MCQ exam as early as possible by going through MCQs.
    - My advice, once you finish a chapter, let us say gall-bladder disease, go through the MCQs in the said chapter. Set your room and alarm as if you are in a real exam.
    - Answer all MCQs in that chapter and keep track of your time spent for each MCQ.
    - After you finish, check your answer and go through the explanation of each question.
    - This approach has several benefits:
        - You know what they focus on in each topic.
        - Recognize your weakness in each topic.
        - Practice multiple times. Just like when you go to play an important soccer game, you practice for a couple of weeks so that you are ready for the big game.
        - Excellent revision.

It is very important to know that just reading books and lecture notes DOES NOT prepare you for the MCQ exam. It needs special preparation, not like any essay **exam**.

Relaxation

- Avoid caffeine-containing drinks especially energy drinks.

- Go to bed early. NEVER EVER go to your exam without a good sleep at night.
- My advice: go and watch a movie early afternoon the day before the exam.
- Try to stop studying during the day before exam (few hours will not be of added benefit). Your brain needs at least twenty-four hours of no INPUT and good SLEEP to consolidate the information.

Avoid Unnecessary Stress

- Go and visit the exam location if it is new to you. It is pre-ferred to go there few days before the exam date at the same time of your exam to see how the traffic is, any road detour, parking area, and exam hall location.
- Get all your documents and tools ready as per exam requirement.
- Go to bed early, wake up early. and go to your exam early.
- Do not consume too much caffeine-containing drinks, dress well, and have a sweater with you (exam hall is cold and your body will be in hyper-sympathetic status).
- Make sure you leave your phone in your car, or if they have a locker, use it to leave your stuff.
- If the exam is long and has a resting period between ses-sions, bring a light meal.
- Read exam instructions well and START YOUR EXAM!

PUZZLE III
INTRA-EXAM STRATEGY

GENERAL PRINCIPLES

When the Exam Is Stable: You Can Out-SMARTS It

On a regular day and a regular exam, you just started answering your MCQs. Both you and the test paper are in a stable condition. In this nice condition, you should out-**SMARTS** the exam, which is an acronym **for**:

S: Stem first

You should read the stem first and carefully. Pay attention to the question asked at the end of the stem. For example, is the question asking about the definitive or initial **treatment?**

M: Mask the options

Once you finished reading the stem, DO NOT start reading the options. Instead, hide the **options**.

A: Anticipate the answer

After hiding the options, anticipate the best correct answer. This step can be done easily with good constructed **MCQ**.

R: Read carefully

It is a must to read both the stem and the options carefully because some options will start with correct sentence and then will end with a totally wrong **sentence.**

T: Tick the anticipated answer

Once you find you anticipated answer, tick it and move on. Do not try to over think **it.**

S: Sixty seconds for each question

Train yourself not to spend more than sixty seconds in answering each question. This skill can be easily acquired by practice. You have to go through pretests before your exam, that is, get any MCQs book and select one section of MCQ and use a timer to go answer them like in a real exam. After you finish answering all questions, look at the answer key and go through the explanations. By this, you hit three birds by one stone, which mean you identify your weaknesses, you do a quick but focused revision of that topic, and warm up for the real **exam.**

EXAMIC SHOCK: ADVANCED MCQ LIFE SUPPORT (AMLS)

Imagine you are following the out-SMARTS strategy and reached the letter "A" for the anticipated answer and then you searched for it but could not find it. You will develop what we call an "examic shock," which is manifested with light heading, sweating, tremor, tachycardia, tachypnea, and near-death feeling. This indicates that the condition is becoming UNSTABLE. Here comes the AMLS guideline to save the exam. You should follow the well-known steps used in resuscitation unstable patient, which is **"ABC"** protocol. In the AMLS situation, we have added more steps, **"ABCDEFHGI"**:

ABCDEFGHI for Unstable MCQ Exam

A: Absolute words and **A**ll or None of the above

There is no always, never, or only in medicine or even in life. Distractors start with these words are usually wrong. "All of the above" option is usually correct especially when you find more than one distractor is correct. Nowadays, it is not common to use absolute words in constructing exam question, but if you see one, you know how to answer it. For example:

Question: Which of the following football club is located in Spain?

> A. Valencia
> B. Sevilla
> C. Deportivo
> D. All of the above
> E. None of the above

Answer: D

B: Best guess

You are ONLY allowed to use it when all strategies fail and when there is no penalty for wrong answers. The theory that explains why your first guess is most likely correct is that your brain has identified the correct answer but could not locate the file where it has been stored. Therefore, NEVER change you first guess UNLESS you remember the correct answer clearly. A study reported that if you depend on your guessing to answer more than four MCQs, your chance to score more than 70% drops from 6% to <2%. This indicates that guessing should be your last strategy to **use**.

C: Comprehensive option and (C) option

Usually, the comprehensive (sounds scientific) option is correct. It does not make sense that the examiner constructs a comprehensive option to be wrong because it is difficult. A funny fact that when examiners place the correct option, they unintentionally try to hide it by putting the option in the middle of the distractors, that is, option (C) or (D). For example:

Question: A 48-year-old female patient with established small bowel obstruction. Which of the following findings will be seen on plain and upright abdominal radiographs?

- A. Marked cecal dilatation
- B. Peripheral gas distribution
- C. Free air under diaphragm
- D. Distended small bowel identifiable by the valvulae conniventes
- E. Prominent haustration in the wall

Answer: D (strategy used: knowledge, comprehensive and "C" option, and repeated words in the stem and the correct option—see H and I strategy further in the book)

D: Double negative and Don't change answers

Double negative gives you positive one. Using the words "not uncommon" is commonly used to give you the sense that it is not common when you go through the sentence quickly. When using the double negative in an option, it is usually correct. **DO NOT** change your answer. Once you answer the question, move on and never think about it. Anecdotally, I had an MCQ exam, and I had answered four MCQs by guessing and then I changed two of them at the end of the exam. Interesting enough, for the two MCQs that I had changed, the new answers were wrong. So, NEVER change your answers. For **example:**

Question: What is correct about medical school graduates worldwide?

- A. Graduates selecting surgery as a career is not uncommon
- B. All graduates get matched in residency program
- C. Medical students never leave medical school until they graduate
- D. Number of applicants to enter medical school is increasing dramatically over the last few years

Answer: A (strategy used: double negative)

E: Extended option (longest), Echo options, and Elimination strategy

Extended (long sentence) option is usually correct especially if it sounds scientific and located in (C) or (D) option. Two options opposite to each other gives you a hint that one of them should be correct. This is called "Echo options." One of the most common-used strategy is the Elimination (exclusion) strategy. Usually, you end up having two options, one of them is correct. By this approach, you increased your chance to get the correct answer from 20–25% to 50%. For example, for Extended and Echo **options**:

Question: A 35-year-old male patient with Crohn's disease present with large output from an enterocutaneous fistula. What is the most likely metabolic changes associated with this fistula?

- A. Hypokalemic metabolic alkalosis
- B. Hypokalemic metabolic acidosis due to HCO3 loss
- C. Hyponatremic metabolic acidosis
- D. Hypercalcemic metabolic alkalosis

Answer: B (strategy used: knowledge, longest option, and echo options "B is echo to C")

F: Funny and Fake options

Sometimes, the examiner writes MCQs with a very funny or fake option. I am sure that at least one MCQ in the exam everyone went through had a laugh or even smile because you felt that the one who created the MCQ is HIGH or trying to be funny. Those funny options or the ones that sound fake are usually wrong because it does not make sense according to our knowledge. For **example**:

Question: What kind of formula would you use to calculate fluid requirement in burn patients?

    A. Texas formula
    B. California formula
    C. New York formula
    D. Washington DC formula
    E. Parkland Formula

Answer: E (strategy used: knowledge, fake and funny option, plus they are all American states, except Parkland)

G: Grammatical clues

If the stem ends with the indefinite article, for example, "an," then the correct response probably begins with a vowel. This unintentional clue is rarely used but if you saw it, then it is a gift for you! For **example**:

Question: Car company that manufacture car brand "Lotus" was established in a:

    A. Italian city
    B. Indian city
    C. American city
    D. British city

Answer: D

H and I: Hidden Internal clues

Always pay attention to the repeated word/sentence in the stem and in the answer, especially if a word is repeated couple of times in the options. This indicates that this word is correct, but you have to look at each distractor that has this repeated word. This could be the hidden clue, and usually, the examiner will write it without paying attention to it. For example:

Question: A 10-year-old boy ingested an open safety pin. Serial abdominal exam is normal. X-ray showed the pin in ileum. What would be the best management option?

    A. Laxative
    B. Serial abdominal X-ray
    C. Urgent endoscopy removal
    D. Laparoscopic removal

Answer: B (strategy used: knowledge, repeated words in the stem and the correction option—Hidden clue)

PUZZLE IV
POST-EXAM STRATEGY

GENERAL PRINCIPLES

There are two scenarios how the exam will end. First, you managed to answer all the MCQs using your knowledge and/or using one or more of the strategies. In this case, make sure you answered all the questions, and you did not miss any questions. If you are using the answer (bubble) sheet to write your answer, make sure you marked all the answers in your answer sheet and make sure you wrote all your personal information in the answer sheet. Second, which is a bad ending, you ran out of time and still have few questions to answer! In this case, you must follow a DAMAGE CONTROL strategy because both you and your exam are about to **arrest!**

THE EXAM IS ABOUT TO ARREST: WHAT TO DO?

You ran out of time and still have some questions to answer. You have to bail out with minimal loss. You have to follow DAMAGE CONTROL strategy (Figure 11). We use this strategy when we have a critical patient in the operating room, and we would like to stop the bleeding or control contamination and close the abdomen to send the patient to the ICU quickly. You have to do the minimal that fails the best and come out with least possible loss. In this exam situation, you have to select one option (I prefer either option "C" or "D") and answer all the remaining questions by selecting one option. DO NOT think, just tick and keep moving; otherwise, your exam is going to die on you. NEVER jump between options (e.g. one question, you select option "C" and the second one "D" and so on). This strategy will probably give you 25% change to answer all the remaining questions **correctly**.

PUZZLE V
RECOVERY STRATEGY

GENERAL PRINCIPLES

At this stage, you finished, and you left the exam area. Is there any strategy to follow? Hell, yes! This stage is critical especially if you have another exam to follow. There are things you must do, and there are traps you SHOULD NOT fall in.

Strategies to Be Followed

You should not be worried about something you have no control on it. You have finished your exam, so you should stop thinking about the exam and move on. This is very important especially if you have another exam to follow. Another strategy is to reward yourself by going out to watch movie or have a nice dinner with friends or family. Some people like to go to the spa for relaxation and massage. The point is DO NOT think of the exam and go back to your normal daily **life**.

Traps You Should NOT Fall in

Never every try to discuss the exam and cross-check your answers. All of us feel that we have to go back to the book and check whether we have our answers correct to feel better. You will be DISAPPOINTED. It has happened to me many times. In several exams, most of my colleagues answered the same question differently. I started feeling bad and down. So, I decided to research for the correct answer. I spent hours going through books and articles. At the end, it turned out that my answer was the correct one. This scenario had a happy ending, but you may not always find a source that tells you whether your or their answer is correct. You will be caught in a vicious circle, which will consume you from inside out. There is a worse scenario than this. If your exam is divided in two parts (e.g. USMLE) separated by few minutes' break and after you finish the first part, you are still thinking about few questions from the earlier paper in the break, which you continue to think about in the second part of the exam as well, then imagine what will happen to the rest of the exam. YOU WILL KILL YOUR EXAM, and you will not be able to resuscitate it.

PUZZLE VI
POST-READING MCQ EXAM

WHAT TO DO NOW?

Now, you have finished reading this book. I hope you enjoyed it! You have to go through the same questions and try to re-answer them by following one or more of the strategies you learned through this book. If you use your knowledge to answer the question, try not to change it because it will reduce your marks. Use the table you created previously to mark your pre-reading MCQ exam. Once you finish answering the post-reading MCQs, look at the changes you made to each question and see whether your mark has changed or not. There are three **possibilities**:

First possibility: your mark DID improve, which means you changed the answer by using one or more of the above-mentioned strategies.

Second possibility: your mark Didn't change, which means you either used your knowledge or you used one or more of the strategies you knew before reading this book and did not know that you are following a certain strategy.

Third possibility: your mark got WORSE, which means that you answered the questions by using your knowledge and then you changed the answer by following one or more of the strategies you learned after reading this book. A major lesson should be learned here. NEVER use one of the strategies when you have the KNOWLEDGE to answer the question. REMEMBER, the aim of this book is to help you answer the MCQ exam when your knowledge does not help you improve your score.

POST-READING 10 MCQS

1.What is the capital of Mexico?

    A. Rio de Janeiro

    B. Veracruz

    C. Ciudad de México

    D. Tabasco City

    E. Salvador

2. Sentinelese is a ward used to describe a

    A. Ancient animal

    B. Tribe

    C. Isolated island

    D. Irish family existed in the past

    E. Organized community in South America

3. Which of the following countries lie on the Equator?

    A. Panama

    B. India

    C. Democratic Republic of the Congo

    D. United Arab of Emirate

    E. Malaysia

4. What would be the most common cause of malpractice suits against physicians?

    A. Failure to diagnose is not uncommon

    B. Incorrect surgery

    C. Errors in medication administration

    D. Poor documentation

    E. Failure to treat

5. What is correct about Paris Saint Germain football club?

    A. Always win the cup

    B. Red-Blue uniform

    C. Never disappoint his fans

    D. Red-Black uniform

    E. Originally from Monte Carlo

6. Which of the following own an island in the Caribbean?

    A. France

    B. United Kingdom

    C. United States of America

    D. All of the above

    E. None of the above

7. Which are the main gases present in the Sun?

    A. Hydrogen and Argon

    B. Oxygen and Carbon dioxide

    C. Nitrogen and Carbon monoxide

    D. Hydrogen and Helium

    E. Nitrogen oxide

8. According to the Occupational Safety and Health Administration (OSHA), informational safety sheets must be present in art rooms that contain which of the following safety risks?

    A. Sharp objects

    B. Loud noises

    C. Heat-producing machinery

    D. Visual hazard

    E. Hazardous and risky chemicals

9. Which of the following are components of Central Processing Unit (CPU) in your computer?

    A. Mouse and monitor

    B. Control unit and USP outlets

    C. Arithmetic logic unit and control unit

    D. Keyboard and mouse

    E. Integrated circuits

10. Which of the following has/have pyramids?

    A. Sudan

    B. Mexico

    C. Italy

    D. Both B and C

    E. All A, B, and C

Answer Key: 1 – C, 2 – B, 3 – C, 4 – A, 5 – B, 6 – D, 7 – D, 8 – E, 9 – C, 10 – E

PUZZLE VII
SYSTEM-BASED REVIEW MCQ

GENERAL PRINCIPLES

This chapter will focus on commonly used MCQs in different surgical specialties. There will be different levels of difficulties to help medical students and residents to understand how the MCQ exam will look like and how to prepare for it. The answers will be provided at the end of each section. My advice is to set a stopwatch for each section and give each question about sixty seconds and go through them like you are in a real exam and then check you answer at the end. Majority of the questions need your knowledge to answer, but if your knowledge failed you, you could use one or more of the strategies you learned from reading this **book**.

PRINCIPLES OF GENERAL SURGERY

1. A 71-year-old male patient is booked for an elective inguinal hernia repair. He has a past medical history of myocadiac infarction (MI) two years ago and chronic atrial fibrillation. What would be the reason to delay his operation?

    A. ECG shows old inferior MI
    B. Mild ankle swelling at the end of the day
    C. Decompensated congestive heart failure
    D. Atrial fibrillation with a heart rate of 88

2. A 65-year-old male patient with recently diagnosis of metastatic colon cancer on chemotherapy. He underwent a palliative left hemicolectomy to relief bowel obstruction. Day 6th postoperatively, he developed refractory shock. A chest X-ray is normal. ECG reveals sinus tachycardia. Of note, a pre-operative ECG was normal. First set of cardiac enzymes was negative. A bedside 2D echo reveals right ventricular strain. What is the most likely diagnosis?

    A. Acute pulmonary embolism
    B. Hypovolemic shock
    C. Septic shock
    D. Acute myocardial infarction leading to cardiogenic shock

3. What is the most effective way to control infection in the hospital?

    A. Proper use of prophylactic antibiotics
    B. Six steps of handwashing
    C. Shaving of the operative site using clipper on OR table
    D. The use of disposable single-use globes

4. **A 57-year-old male patient was intubated and admitted to the ICU in severe sepsis and coagulopathy two days after laparotomy for perforated appendix. On Day 5, he developed bloody aspirate in the nasogastric tube with melena. What would be the most likely diagnosis in this patient?**

   A. Ruptured AV malformation

   B. Dieulafoy's lesion

   C. Mallory–Weiss syndrome

   D. Stress ulceration

5. **On postoperative Day 6, an otherwise healthy 55-year-old male patient recovering from open cholecystectomy is noted to have a fever of 38.6°C. Which of the following is the most common nosocomial infection postoperatively?**

   A. Surgical site infection

   B. Urinary tract infection

   C. Hospital acquired pneumonia

   D. Intravenous catheter-related infection

6. **A surgical resident is about to consent a 29-year-old patient for open appendectomy. The patient refused to sign and wants to be managed conservatively despite full explanation. The patient is fully awake and oriented. What would be the appropriate action?**

   A. Ask for hospital committee to make the decision

   B. Refer the patient to another hospital

   C. Observe him and if he got worse and confused, then take to OR as emergency case

   D. Respect patient's will

7. Four days after uneventful cholecystectomy, an asymptomatic middle-aged female patient is found to have a serum sodium level of 125 mEq/L (normal 135–145 mEq/L). She has been in clear fluid diet for this period. Which of the following is the most appropriate initial management strategy for this patient?

   A. Administer hypertonic saline solution
   B. Restriction of free water
   C. Aggressive diuresis with furosemide
   D. Oral replacement with sodium chloride tablet

8. A 50-year-old homeless male patient was brought to the ER in a stupors state. Blood pressure is 100/50 mmHg, heart rate 120 beats/minute, respiratory rate 35/minute, and his temperature is 40°C. He was found to have cellulitis of his left foot. Below are his lab results: Na+ 150 mEq/L (135–145), K+ 2.5 mEq/L (3.5–5.0), pH 7.2 (7.35–7.45), PCO2 25 mmHg (35–45), HCO3 10 mEq/L (24–26). What is the acid–base status?

   A. Metabolic acidosis and metabolic alkalosis
   B. Respiratory acidosis with partial metabolic compensation
   C. Metabolic acidosis with partial respiratory compensation
   D. Respiratory acidosis

Answer Key: 1 – C, 2 – A, 3 – B, 4 – D, 5 – A, 6 – D, 7 – B, 8 – C

HEAD AND NECK

1. **A 20-year-old female patient presents with a painful lump in the midline of her neck below her chin. The lump is red, firm, tender, measures 1 cm, no discharge, and moves on tongue protrusion. What would be the best initial treatment option?**

    A. Antibiotic and observation
    B. Fine needle aspiration
    C. Incision and drainage
    D. Sistrunk procedure

2. **A 66-year-old smoker male patient presents with pain-less lateral neck swelling. FNA showed squamous cell carcinoma. All initial investigations like neck/chest CT and panendoscopy were inconclusive. What is the best next step?**

    A. Radiotherapy
    B. Tonsillectomy
    C. Lateral neck dissection
    D. Bilateral neck dissection

3. **A 60-year-old smoker male patient presents with pain-less left swelling over the angle of the mandible. CT neck showed well-defined lesion in the superficial part of the parotid gland. FNA was inconclusive twice. What is the best next step?**

    A. Tru-cut biopsy
    B. Incisional biopsy
    C. Enucleation
    D. Superficial parotidectomy

4. **A 70-year-old male patient underwent right superficial parotidectomy for pleomorphic adenoma. Few weeks later, he presented to the clinic complaining of sweating when he talks or thinks about food. What is the most likely explanation?**

    A. Obstruction of the main parotid gland duct
    B. Injury to auriculotemporal nerve
    C. Neuropraxia of one of the facial nerve branches
    D. Deep-seated infected seroma

Answer Key: 1 – A, 2 – B, 3 – D, 4 – B

ESOPHAGUS

1. A 63-year-old male patient is admitted to the emergency department five days after a laparoscopic Heller myotomy for achalasia with fever, chills, and epigastric and left shoulder pain. His temperature is 39°C, white blood cell (WBC) count is 22,000/μL, and hemoglobin is 15 g/dL. A computed tomography (CT) scan shows a left subphrenic fluid collection and left lower lobe consolidation. What is the cause of the clinical scenario?

    A. Left lower lobe pneumonia
    B. Distal esophageal perforation
    C. Hematoma from splenic capsule injury
    D. Hematoma from short gastric vessel

2. A 55-year-old patient with a long history of a gastro-esophageal reflux disease had an endoscopic examination and biopsy of the lower esophagus. Histology report showed intestinal metaplasia. Treatment is indicated to minimize the risk of developing which type of esophageal cancer?

    A. Adenocarcinoma
    B. Squamous cell carcinoma
    C. Lymphoma
    D. Gastrointestinal stromal tumor (GIST)

3. A 41-year-old male patient complains of regurgitation of saliva and undigested food. Barium swallow and manometry were done. What would be diagnostic for achalasia in manometry?

    A. Absence of peristalsis
    B. Loss of relaxation
    C. Lower esophageal sphincter pressure of 20 mmHg
    D. Uncoordinated contraction

4. **A 58-year-old otherwise healthy female patient is diagnosed with achalasia with megaesophagus, based on history and manometry finding. She underwent pneumatic dilatation which was complicated with free perforation based on CT scan. She is hemodynamically stable. What would be the best treatment option?**

    A. Conservative treatment with NPO and antibiotic
    B. Esophageal stenting
    C. Surgical repair of perforation and myotomy
    D. Esophagectomy

5. **A 64-year-old otherwise healthy male patient presents to the clinic with heartburn and regurgitation for six months. Initial investigation revealed anemia only. What is the most crucial management option?**

    A. Proton pump inhibitor for two weeks and then reassess
    B. Upper GI series
    C. Esophagogastroduodenoscopy
    D. 24-h pH monitor to diagnose gastroesophageal reflux

6. **A 54-year-old otherwise healthy male patient is diagnosed as a case of symptomatic type III paraesophageal hiatus hernia with short esophagus based on clinical, imaging, and endoscopy. What is the best treatment option?**

    A. Fundoplication with Collis' gastroplasty
    B. Toupet fundoplication
    C. Transthoracic closure of the defect and then fundoplication
    D. Transabdominal hernia closure with magnetic sphincter augmentation device placement

7. A 60-year-old male patient is diagnosed as early distal esophageal adenocarcinoma. Histopathology showed T1b cancer. Metastatic workup did not show any sign of lymph node or distal metastases. What is the best treatment option?

    A. Neoadjuvant chemoradiation followed by resection
    B. Endoscopic mucosal resection (EMR)
    C. Distal esophagectomy
    D. Near/total esophagectomy

8. A 71-year-old female patient underwent transhiatal total esophagectomy for stage III esophageal cancer post neoadjuvant chemoradiation. Seven days postoperative, she came back to the ER with dyspnea and palpitation with tachycardia but stable blood pressure. Initial work up revealed elevated WBC with C-reactive protein, and chest radiography showed left pleural effusion. What is the most important initial step in management?

    A. NPO, IV fluid, and antibiotics
    B. Urgent esophagogram with barium contrast
    C. Urgent CT chest and abdomen with contrast to rule out esophageal perforation
    D. Urgent chest tube and send fluid for analysis and culture

Answer Key: 1 – B, 2 – A, 3 – A, 4 – D, 5 – C, 6 – A, 7 – D, 8 – A

ABDOMINAL WALL AND CAVITY

1. **A 58-year-old female patient on aspirin for TIA presents to the ER with sudden pain in the right lower quadrant after coughing associated with low-grade fever, anorexia, and nausea. On examination, stable hemodynamic. There is a tender mass in the right lower quadrant with muscular spasm. White blood count of 11,000. CT with IV contrast shows an apparent mass in the abdominal wall. What is the best treatment option?**

    A. Reverse the effect of aspirin and discharge
    B. Admit for analgesia and observation
    C. Incision and drainage with IV antibiotics
    D. Urgent diagnostic laparoscopic

2. **A 38-year-old female patient underwent right hemicolectomy for large colonic polyp. On the sixth day, the patient starts complaining of pain in the wound, and when you examined the patient, you found a serosanguinous fluid coming from the incision. What is the best treatment option?**

    A. Daily wet dressing
    B. Remove staples and start IV antibiotic
    C. Urgent CT abdomen with contrast to rule out anastomotic leak
    D. Take the patient to the operation room

3. **A 24-year-old male patient presents with postprandial chronic abdominal pain. He is healthy and never had surgery. CT abdomen showed picture of left sided paraduodenal mesocolic hernia. What is the most important step in hernia repair?**

    A. Right lateral to medial visceral rotation
    B. Incision of the peritoneal attachment just right to IMV
    C. Kocher procedure
    D. Left lateral to medial visceral rotation

4. **A 45-year-old male patient presents with severe right abdominal pain with nausea. On exam, he is tachycardic but stable blood pressure with mild tenderness over right side of abdomen but no mass. Initial investigation revealed mild leukocytosis, and rest of blood tests are normal. Abdominal US was normal, but CT scan showed only inflamed omentum. What is the best next step?**

    A. Observation and analgesia
    B. Oral cholecystogram
    C. Conventional mesenteric angiogram
    D. Exploratory laparotomy

5. **A 62-year-old male patient presents to clinic with mild abdominal pain and constitutional symptoms with decreased urination. Examination only showed mild generalized discomfort on palpation. Initial investigation showed elevation of ESR and C-reactive protein. CT abdomen finding is suggestive of retroperitoneal fibrosis with bilateral mild hydronephrosis. What is the most crucial next step?**

    A. Steroid and immunosuppressant
    B. MRI with contrast
    C. Double J ureteric stents
    D. CT-guided Tru-cut biopsy

6. **A 70-year-old lady presents to the ER with abdominal pain and vomiting for twenty-four hours. Pulse is 100/minute, BP 100/70 mm Hg, and temperature 38°C. Abdomen is distended with mild tenderness all over, and bowel sounds are exaggerated with a tender tense swelling in the left groin and absent cough impulse. What would be the most appropriate management?**

    A. Apply warm compresses over the swelling while in Trendelenburg position

    B. Attempt reduction under sedation in the operating room

    C. Groin exploration

    D. Exploratory laparotomy

7. **A 75-year-old female patient presents to the ER with cramping abdominal pain and vomiting for the past six hours. She never had surgery, but she has been treated for chronic inner thigh pain for six months. Abdomen is distended with diffuse tenderness and exaggerated bowel sound. Groin exam is normal. What is the most likely diagnosis?**

    A. Obturator hernia

    B. Psoas abscess

    C. Pott's disease

    D. Dissection abdominal aortic aneurysm

8. **As a surgeon examining the inguinal region of a patient, the inguinal ligament will be a key landmark. Which structure is the origin of this ligament?**

    A. Superficial abdominal fascia

    B. Internal abdominal muscle

    C. External oblique aponeurosis

    D. Transversus abdominis

9. **You were called urgently to see a patient with severe thigh pain in recovery room just recovered from anesthesia post laparoscopic right inguinal hernia repair for pantaloon hernia. What is the most likely injured nerve?**

    A. Femoral branch of the genitofemoral
    B. Lateral femoral cutaneous
    C. Iliohypogastric
    D. Ilioinguinal

10. **A 60-year-old male patient will undergo repair of the inguinal hernia. The patient is concerned about the outcome and complication of surgery. Which of the following statements should be explained to the patient?**

    A. 10% recurrence rate is acceptable in general
    B. Herniorrhaphy is the preferred approach
    C. Loss of his testicle is very likely
    D. Postoperative wound infection is 2%

11. **A 65-year-old female patient was brought to the ER with abdominal pain, vomiting, and abdominal distension for thirty-eight hours, one-year post laparotomy for perforated duodenal ulcer. Examination reveals pulse of 100 min, BP 100/75 mmHg, and temperature 37.9°C. Abdomen is distended with a tender 6 × 8 cm tense swelling at the lower end of a mid-line scar. WBC count was 12,500, Hb 13.3 g/ dL, K 3.1, Na 134, and ABG showed metabolic acidosis. Abdominal X-rays showed dilated bowel loops. CXR and ECG are normal. What is the most appropriate next step?**

    A. Urgent CT abdomen with oral and IV contrast
    B. Urgent laparotomy after resuscitation
    C. NPO, resuscitation, HCO3, and monitoring
    D. IV antibiotic and urgent incision and drainage with debridement

12. **The on-call surgical team took a 55-year-old female patient with irreducible tender right femoral hernia to the OR for emergent groin exploration and repair. After induction, the hernia was reduced spontaneously. What would be the best approach now?**

    A. Make your incision over the hernia and use a grasper to pull out the bowel to assess viability

    B. Proceed with McVay repair

    C. Use an absorbable mesh for repair

    D. Convert to midline laparotomy

13. **A 71-year-old male patient presents to the clinic with recurrent right inguinal hernia, six months post transabdominal preperitoneal (TAPP) laparoscopic mesh repair. What would be the best operative option?**

    A. Laparoscopic total extraperitoneal repair (TEP)

    B. Laparoscopic extended TEP (e-TEP)

    C. Open mesh repair

    D. Open Stoppa mesh repair

14. **An elderly male patient with a large indirect inguinal hernia was admitted for elective repair. At groin exploration, a firm, cord-like structure was divided accidentally. What would be the best option?**

    A. Call the urologist and document

    B. Approximate both ends using 5.0 absorbable monofilament suture

    C. Approximate both ends and repair over a stent

    D. Leave the two ends, insert a drain, and then close the wound

15. A slightly overweight (BMI = 32) 49-year-old male patient underwent open sigmoid colectomy for diverticular disease five years ago. Now, he has asymptomatic ventral incisional hernia in the upper part of his incision that measures 5 × 4 cm. What is the best treatment option?

    A. Watchful waiting because he is asymptomatic

    B. Application of abdominal binder with close follow-up

    C. Open repair with onlay mesh and drains insertion

    D. Laparoscopic mesh repair

16. A 25-year-old healthy female patient presents with umbilical hernia with about 2.5-cm defect. Which of the following technique has the lowest recurrent rate?

    A. Interrupted nonabsorbable suture primary repair

    B. Sublay mesh repair

    C. Inlay mesh repair

    D. Only mesh repair

Answer Key: 1 – B, 2 – D, 3 – B, 4 – A, 5 – D, 6 – C, 7 – A, 8 – C, 9 – B, 10 – D, 11 – B, 12 – D, 13 – C, 14 – A, 15 – D, 16 – B

STOMACH AND DUODENUM

1. **A 59-year-old lady who's on diclofenac for osteoarthritis came to the ER with a one-day history of hematemesis and melena. Her hemoglobin level was 9 g/dL. The bleeding was controlled on upper GI endoscopy. Which of the following is associated with the highest risk for recurrent bleeding from a peptic ulcer?**

    A. Visible vessel within the ulcer
    B. Presence of erythematous mucosa surrounding the ulcer
    C. Presence of blood clots in the stomach
    D. A black spot in the ulcer's base

2. **A 59-year-old male patient presents with repeated vomiting for few days. He has been treated for gastric ulcer with PPI for one year. Initial workup revealed picture of gastric outlet obstruction. What is the best initial management?**

    A. Antrectomy and Billroth II reconstruction
    B. Gastrojejunostomy with feeding jejunostomy
    C. Urgent endoscopic decompression and biopsy to rule out cancer
    D. NPO, NGT, IV fluid, and PPI

3. **A 65-year-old female patient underwent urgent EGD and clipping of a bleeding duodenal ulcer. 24 hours post procedure, she developed hematemesis. After fluid administration, what is the best next option?**

    A. CT angiogram to localize the bleeder
    B. Repeat endoscopy in OR
    C. Conventional angiogram with embolization
    D. Exploratory laparotomy and oversaw the bleeder

4. **A 48-year-old male patient presented to the ER in shock with rigid abdomen. He was taken to the OR for laparotomy after initial workup. Intraoperatively, a 4-cm perforated gastric ulcer in the antrum was identified with gross contamination with unstable hemodynamics. What would be the best treatment for this ulcer?**

    A. Omental patch after taking biopsy to rule out cancer
    B. Gastrostomy through the defect and come out
    C. Distal gastrectomy with Billroth II reconstruction
    D. Distal gastrectomy with Roux-en-Y reconstruction

5. **A 59-year-old male patient underwent EGD for vague abdominal pain, anorexia, and weight loss. Endoscopy showed fungating mass in the body of the stomach. Biopsies were taken, which showed adenocarcinoma penetrating the subserosa. Endoscopic US and CT scan did not show any extragastric extension. What is the best next treatment option?**

    A. Neoadjuvant therapy
    B. Endoscopic mucosal resection
    C. Subtotal gastrectomy with jejunogastrostomy
    D. Total gastrectomy with Roux-en-Y jejunal interposition

6. **An elderly female patient was diagnosed with adenocarcinoma of the proximal stomach. What is the method of choice to assess depth of invasion?**

    A. CT abdomen with IV contrast
    B. MRI abdomen
    C. Endoscopic ultrasound
    D. PET scan

7. **A 69-year-old male patient presents with hematemesis to the ER. After resuscitation, he was admitted to the ICU for monitoring. Endoscopy was performed, which revealed a bleeding ulcer over an exophytic lesion in the antrum. Biopsy showed normal gastric cells. What would be the most useful tool for diagnosis?**

> A. CT scan with oral and IV contrast
> B. Percutaneous CT-guided biopsy
> C. Repeat endoscopy with deeper biopsy
> D. Laparoscopic wedge resection

8. **A 51-year-old female patient presents to ER with sudden abdominal pain and persistent vomiting. On examination, stable hemodynamics with mild tender fullness in the epigastric area. Initial work up and imaging suggests gastric bezoar. What is the initial treatment option?**

> A. NPO, NGT, and IV fluid and observation because majority will pass the stomach spontaneously
> B. Enzymatic and soda therapies
> C. Endoscopic fragmentation
> D. Gastrotomy and removal of bezoar

Answer Key: 1 – A, 2 – D, 3 – B, 4 – B, 5 – A, 6 – C, 7 – A, 8 – B

GALLBLADDER AND BILIARY TREE

1. **A 39-year-old female patient complains of jaundice and RUQ discomfort six days after cholecystectomy. Her vital signs are within normal, and there is RUQ tenderness. WBC count is 11,000/mL. Total bilirubin 6 mg/dL and direct bilirubin 5 mg/dL. What is the most appropriate next step in management?**

    A. Abdominal ultrasound
    B. HIDA scan
    C. MRCP
    D. PTC

2. **A 42-year-old male patient, known case of gallstone, underwent ERCP for choledocholithiasis. What is the next most appropriate step in management?**

    A. Discharge home and follow-up in the clinic
    B. MRCP to confirm the absence of complication
    C. Repeat ERCP after two weeks to confirm the clearance of CBD
    D. Perform cholecystectomy on the same admission

3. **A 39-year-old female patient complains of jaundice and RUQ discomfort six days after cholecystectomy. Stable vital signs with RUQ tenderness. WBC count is 12,000/mL, and serum Total bilirubin level is 4 mg/dL. Ultrasound reveals a 10 × 10 cm sub-hepatic fluid collection with normal caliber of the CBD and intrahepatic biliary ducts. What is the next most appropriate step in management?**

    A. ERCP
    B. PTC and stent insertion
    C. Ultrasound-guided percutaneous drainage
    D. Exploratory laparotomy and peritoneal lavage

4. **A 49-year-old lady, post gastric bypass for morbid obesity two years ago, is transferred to the ICU with hypotension and decreased level of consciousness after being admitted with a three-day history of RUQ abdominal pain, high-grade fever with chills, and jaundice. Ultrasound reveals dilated CBD and intra-hepatic biliary ducts. No gastroenterologist or interventional radiologist is available. What is the next most appropriate step in management?**

    A. Cholecystostomy tube insertion
    B. Choledochotomy and T-tube insertion
    C. Cholecystectomy and common bile duct (CBD) exploration
    D. Cholecystectomy with intra-operative cholangiography

5. **A 45-year-old female patient with sickle cell anemia underwent laparoscopic cholecystectomy for recurrent biliary colic. What would be the most comment type of stones in this patient?**

    A. Black
    B. Brown
    C. Cholesterol
    D. Mixed

6. **A 38-year-old female patient is admitted to the hospital with two-day history of RUQ pain and nausea. Initial work up showed leukocytosis, and US abdomen thickened gallbladder with impacted 2 × 2 cm stone in gallbladder neck. What is the best management option?**

    A. HIDA scan to confirm the diagnosis
    B. Conservative therapy with NPO, analgesia, and IV antibiotic
    C. Percutaneous cholecystostomy
    D. Urgent laparoscopic cholecystectomy

7. You're assessing a 60-year-old lady with recurrent attacks of biliary colic for the past six months in the surgical clinic. Which of the following is NOT risk factor for gallbladder carcinoma?

    A. Large gallstone of 4 cm
    B. Gallbladder polyp of 0.8 cm
    C. Choledochal cyst
    D. Chronic Salmonella typhi

8. Uneventful laparoscopic cholecystectomy for acute cholecystitis was done for a 60-year-old male patient. The procedure appeared to be straightforward. The patient had smooth recovery initially. The histopathology showed completely resected adenocarcinoma of gallbladder invading muscularis layer. After workup, the patient was labeled as T1b, N0, M0. What is the best treatment option?

    A. Cholecystectomy is enough and need no further therapy
    B. Re-exploration for laparoscopic ports excision
    C. Partial hepatectomy with lymphadenectomy
    D. Trisegmentectomy

Answer Key: 1 – A, 2 – D, 3 – C, 4 – B, 5 – A, 6 – D, 7 – B, 8 – C

LIVER AND PANCREAS

1. **A 49-year-old male patient was admitted to the ICU with severe pancreatitis. Which treatment option was proven to improve outcome in this patient?**

    A. Wide-spectrum IV antibiotics
    B. Fluid resuscitation
    C. Early endoscopic retrograde cholangiopancreatography (ERCP)
    D. Invasive monitoring and inotropic support

2. **During the examination of a 56-year-old male patient with acute hemorrhagic pancreatitis. After resuscitation. What would be your appropriate intervention?**

    A. Endoscopic retrograde cholangiopancreatography (ERCP) with balloon insertion inside the pancreatic duct
    B. Percutaneous intravascular injection of sclerosing agent
    C. Angio-embolization
    D. Laparotomy and packing of lesser sac

3. **After a weekend of heavy meal, a 38-year-old male patient presents with sudden severe abdominal pain and vomiting. Preliminary blood test revealed; hyponatremia and serum amylase of 998 IU. What is the investigative and prognostic modality of choice for your suspected diagnosis?**

    A. Abdominal ultrasound
    B. Abdominal CT scan
    C. Endoscopic retrograde cholangiopancreatography (ERCP)
    D. Magnetic resonance cholangiopancreatography (MRCP)

4. A 60-year-old male patient was admitted with acute pancreatitis. Initial investigation revealed a WBC of 17,000/µL, glucose level of 12 mmol/L, AST of 300 iµ/L, and amylase is 1020 iµ/L. Which one of the factors mentioned above is NOT a prognostic factor for acute pancreatitis?

    A. Patient's age
    B. WBC
    C. AST
    D. Amylase level

5. A 55-year-old male patient treated conservatively as acute pancreatitis following abdominal trauma and discharged after seven days. Two weeks following discharge, he developed abdominal pain and vomiting and was readmitted. During assessment, examination revealed epigastric mass, confirmed by ultrasound and CT scan. Pancreatic pseudocyst is diagnosed. Which of the following complication might occur if this pathology is not managed appropriately?

    A. Bleeding
    B. Malignant transformation
    C. Diabetes mellitus
    D. Anaphylactic shock if ruptured

6. A 48-year-old male patient was admitted with the diagnosis of uncomplicated diverticulitis. Two days later, he spiked high every with upper abdominal pain. He is stable hemodynamic with tenderness in the upper abdomen. Urgent CT scan was performed with showed 5 × 6 cm right liver lobe abscess. What is the optimal treatment option?

    A. Broad-spectrum IV antibiotics
    B. CT-guided percutaneous drainage
    C. Laparoscopic drainage
    D. Open drainage and irrigation through midline incision

7. **A 33-year-old male patient is going to the OR for open drainage of liver hydatid cyst. What is the best approach for preoperative preparation?**

    A. IV steroid to prevent anaphylactic shock if leaked

    B. Percutaneous US-guided intracystic injection of hypertonic saline to neutralize the content before surgical drainage

    C. Albendazole for 7–10 days

    D. Open drainage and irrigation through midline incision

8. **A 25-year-old female patient on oral contraceptive pills presents to the clinic with mild discomfort in the right upper quadrant. CT abdomen with IV contrast revealed hypervascular 2 × 2cm lesion in the left liver lobe with early peripheral enhancement with centripetal progression but NO washout. What is the best treatment option?**

    A. Stop oral contraceptive pill with close follow-up

    B. Angioembolization

    C. Percutaneous radio-frequency ablation

    D. Enucleation

9. **A 38-year-old healthy female patient presents to the clinic with vague upper abdominal pain. Initial work up including CT showed well-defined, 4-cm, thick, irregular single cyst with internal septation and papillary projections. What would be the best treatment option?**

    A. Regular follow-up with clinical and imaging assessment

    B. Fine needle aspiration

    C. Enucleations

    D. Surgical resection

10. A 66-year-old male patient with hepatitis C-induced liver cirrhosis. During regular screening for hepatocellular carcinoma (HCC), US and CT scan showed 2-cm solitary lesion in the right liver lobe suggestive of HCC with elevation of alpha fetoprotein (AFP). What would be the best management option?

    A. Intense follow-up every 3–6 months with CT scan and AFP

    B. Rule out extrahepatic disease

    C. Fine needle aspiration

    D. Anatomical resection

Answer Key: 1 – B, 2 – C, 3 – B, 4 – D, 5 – A, 6 – B, 7 – C, 8 – A, 9 – D, 10 – B

SPLEEN

1. **An 18-year-old male patient, known case of Thalassemia, complains of left upper abdominal pain worse on respiration and radiate to the left scapula on Day 7 post elective splenectomy for hypersplenism. Examination reveals a temperature of 38.6°C, decreased air entry on the left side, and left upper quadrant abdominal tenderness. What is the most likely cause of this condition?**

    A. Retained splenic tissue causing recurrent hypersplenism
    B. Portal vein thrombosis
    C. Pancreatic tail injury
    D. Gastric perforation

2. **There are few indications for splenectomy. Which of the following condition splenectomy is completely curative?**

    A. Hereditary spherocytosis
    B. Idiopathic thrombocytopenic purpura
    C. Chronic myeloid leukemia
    D. Thalassemia major

3. **A 23-year-old female patient has CT abdomen for suspecting appendicitis, which showed just lymphadenitis in the terminal ileum, but there was an incidental distal splenic artery aneurysm. What is the best treatment option?**

    A. Close monitoring until it become symptomatic
    B. Angiogram and stenting
    C. Angioembolization
    D. Splenectomy

4. **A 31-year-old male patient, known case of IV drug addiction, presents to the ER with decreases level of consciousness, fever, and upper abdominal pain for one day with hypotension responding to fluid and marked tenderness in the left upper guardant. Initial work up showed leukocytosis and CT scan showed nonenhanced spleen with air-fluid level with loculation. After resuscitation, what is the best treatment option?**

    A. Splenectomy

    B. Percutaneous drainage

    C. Broad-spectrum antibiotic

    D. Urgent MRI abdomen to confirm the diagnosis

Answer Key: 1 – C, 2 – A, 3 – D, 4 – A

SMALL BOWEL

1. **A 42-year-old female patient is admitted to the emergency department with severe colicky pain, vomiting, and abdominal distention. She has not passed stools or flatus for forty-eight hours. X-rays of the abdomen confirm the presence of small bowel obstruction. What is the most likely cause of bowel obstruction in this patient?**

    A. Hernia

    B. Crohn's disease

    C. Gallstone ileus

    D. Small bowel malrotation with volvulus

2. **A 29-year-old male patient presents with a twenty-four-hour history of abdominal pain and anorexia. Periumbilical pain shifted to the right lower quadrant. He is febrile and has leukocytosis. Examination reveals tenderness of the right lower quadrant and guarding. Laparoscopic evaluation reveals a normal appendix and cecum with a significantly inflamed terminal ileum with fat creeping and lymphadenopathy. Which of the following is the MOST appropriate next step?**

    A. Proceed with appendectomy

    B. Ileocecectomy

    C. Formal right hemicolectomy

    D. Stop the procedure and conservative therapy

3. A 78-year-old male patient is brought to the ER with a twelve-hour history of constant central abdominal pain with nausea and vomiting. He has a history of atrial fibrillation on digoxin. Examination reveals a distended abdomen with tenderness and guarding in the umbilical area and diminished bowel sounds. WBC is 24,000. What is the most appropriate investigation for this patient?

   A. Abdominal ultrasound

   B. CT abdomen with IV contrast

   C. Conventional angiogram

   D. Upper and lower GI endoscopy

4. In a 23-year-old patient with suspected appendicitis, layered densities of fat and soft tissue inside the bowel lumen on CT of the abdomen. What does this finding suggest?

   A. Small bowel volvulus

   B. Appendix mucocele

   C. Intussusception

   D. Meckel's diverticulum

5. **A 37-year-old lady with a history of Cesarean section presents with a three-day history of constipation, abdominal distention, and vomiting. Pulse: 90/minute, BP: 120/55, and Temperature: 37.5°C. The abdomen was diffusely tender and distended but not guarded. Bowel sounds were sluggish, and rectal examination showed an empty rectum. Abdominal X-ray showed dilated small bowel to 3 cm with on free air. What would be the management of this lady in the first 48 hours?**

    A. NGT, intravenous fluid, and correction of electrolyte imbalance

    B. Immediate consideration for parenteral nutrition

    C. Reduction by rectal air insufflation

    D. Immediate exploratory laparotomy

6. **A 37-year-old lady with a history of Cesarean section presents with a three-day history of constipation, abdominal distention, and vomiting. Pulse: 90/minute, BP: 120/55 and Temperature: 37.5°C. The abdomen was diffusely tender and distended but not guarded. Bowel sounds were sluggish, and rectal examination showed an empty rectum. Abdominal X-ray showed dilated small bowel to 3 cm with on free air. What would be the management of this lady in the first 48 hours?**

    A. Vomiting of feculent material

    B. Severe abdominal pain with minimal abdominal findings

    C. Continuous bloody diarrhea with mucus

    D. Absence of gas-filled bowel loops noticed in abdominal plain x-ray

7. **A 53-year-old male patient seen in Emergency Room with severe abdominal pain and vomiting for the past eighteen hours. On abdominal exam, slightly distended and tender mainly in the upper part, blood test showed leukocytosis with hyponatremia. All of the following radiological findings are consistent with mechanical bowel obstruction EXCEPT:**

    A. A "step ladder" pattern
    B. Dilated small bowel loops
    C. Air-fluid levels at uniform height in same bowel loop
    D. Rows of small gas accumulations in valvulae conniventes (strings of pearls)

8. **A 64-year-old male patient seen in ER with recurrent abdominal pain and vomiting for the past three months. He has history of radiotherapy for stage II rectal cancer post low anterior resection six months ago. Surgical team decided to take him for exploratory laparotomy. Intraoperatively, there is extensive dense adhesions in the pelvis incasing a loop of small bowel. What is the best surgical option?**

    A. Release all adhesion to prevent recurrent bowel obstruction
    B. Bypass the entrapped small bowel
    C. Diverting stoma
    D. Resection and anastomosis

9. **A 24-year-old female patient came to the clinic with recurrent perianal small abscess all of them treated conservatively. She brought a stool calprotectin level 920 µg/mg. What is the best next option?**

    A. Reassurance, and it is most likely related to perianal abscess

    B. Repeat stool calprotectin and stool occult blood

    C. Start her on antibiotic and send stool for ovum and parasite

    D. Refer her to gastroenterology for lower GI endoscopy

10. **A 40-year-old female patient, case of severe Crohn's disease, is taken to the OR for strictureplasty. In the OR, 13-cm single chronic fibrotic narrowing of the proximal ileum. What is the most appropriate option?**

    A. Heineke–Mikulicz

    B. Finney

    C. Moskel–Walske–Neumayer

    D. Side-to-side isoperistaltic strictureplasty

11. **A 57-year-old female patient presents to the ER with abdominal pain, diarrhea, and flushing for few days. Abdominal exam was unremarkable. Initial work up revealed CT scan finding of 3-cm dense mesenteric mass with radiating stranding in the ileum. The patient is going to the OR for resection. What is the best approach to prevent crisis related to this lesion that might happen during surgery?**

    A. IV fluid and vasopressor

    B. Broad-spectrum antibiotic

    C. Antihistamine

    D. Somatostatin

12. A 64-year-old male patient, known case of Crohn's disease for 15 years, presents with abdominal pain and vomiting for five days. Abdominal exam showed mild distention with mild tenderness. Rectal exam was positive for bloody stool. Initial work up showed anemia and apple-core lesion in the distal ileum about 5 cm from the ileocecal valve with no other significant finding. What is the best treatment option?

    A. Right hemicolectomy including the involved ileum

    B. Segmental resection with lymphadenectomy

    C. Ileocolic bypass

    D. Neoadjuvant chemotherapy then surgery

Answer Key: 1 – A, 2 – D, 3 – B, 4 – C, 5 – A, 6 – A, 7 – C, 8 – B, 9 – D, 10 – B, 11 – D, 12 – A

APPENDIX

1. **A 21-year-old male patient presents to the ER with six hours history of vague, periumbilical abdominal pain, and anorexia. The pain has shifted to right lower quadrant. On examination, he is found to have tenderness over McBurney point along with rigidity. What is the most likely explanation of changing in the character of pain?**

    A. Inflammation of visceral peritoneum produces localizing pain
    B. Distention of the appendiceal lumen
    C. Unmyelinated fibers carry pain signals with thoracic and lumber spine nerves
    D. Movement of inflamed parietal peritoneum induces rebound tenderness

2. **A 21-year-old pregnant patient in her 35 weeks of gestation presents to the ER with symptoms and signs highly suggestive of acute appendicitis. What is the best operative approach?**

    A. Make your incision over McBurney point
    B. Mark the area of maximum tenderness preoperatively to guide you
    C. Perform appendectomy though lower midline incision
    D. Laparoscopic appendectomy

3. **A 26-year-old married female patient presents with three-day history of right lower quadrant pain and fever. Examination reveals a tender, palpable, right lower quadrant mass. There is no evidence of peritonitis or sepsis. Work up reveals leukocytosis and an inflammatory 5 × 4 cm mass with air-fluid level on ultrasound. What is the best treatment option?**

   A. Conservative therapy with antibiotic
   B. Emergent gynecology consultation for evaluation and treatment of possible ectopic pregnancy
   C. US-guided percutaneous drainage
   D. Urgent appendectomy

4. **A 65-year-old male patient presents to the ER with acute right iliac fossa (RIF) pain. There is a low-grade fever with localized tenderness, guarding, and rebound tenderness in the RIF. His WBC is 11,000 with normal serum amylase level. What is the appropriate next line of management?**

   A. Request a CT scan of the abdomen with IV and oral contrast
   B. Admit and actively observe the patient without analgesia
   C. Discharge the patient on oral antibiotics with close follow-up
   D. Transfer the patient to the OR for urgent surgery

5. **A 45-year-old African worker presents to the ER with back pain, fever, night sweats, and a lump in his right groin. On examination, there is tenderness in the thoracolumbar spin. Abdominal exam reveals fullness in the left iliac fossa and a fluctuant swelling in the femoral triangle with positive cough impulse. What is the most likely diagnosis?**

   A. Femoral artery pseudoaneurysm

   B. Strangulated indirect inguinal hernia

   C. Psoas abscess

   D. Inguinal lymphadenopathy

6. **A 35-year-old patient underwent open appendectomy for perforated appendix. On the fifth postoperative day, the patient develops a brownish, foul-smelling discharge from the wound. This continues with a daily volume of 50–100 mL. What is the most likely diagnosis?**

   A. Wound dehiscence

   B. Appendico-cutaneous fistula

   C. Wound infection/abscess with gas-producing organism

   D. Stitch sinus with granuloma

7. **A 68-year-old patient is taken to the OR for laparoscopic appendectomy. During abdominal exploration, 3-cm mass was identified at the base of the appendix. What is best decision now?**

   A. Proceed with appendectomy and post-operative colonoscopy

   B. Just perform laparoscopic tissue biopsy and send for frozen section

   C. Convert to open appendectomy

   D. Perform formal right hemicolectomy

8. A 55-year-old healthy male patient is taken to the OR for elective open right inguinal hernia repair. Upon opening the hernia sac, gelatinous fluid with whitish spots on the peritoneum. What is the best next step?

    A. Take samples from the fluid and peritoneum and close the wound
    B. Convert to laparoscopic exploration
    C. Convert to formal midline laparotomy
    D. Fix the hernia (hernioplasty) and send the excised sac for pathology

9. A 22-year-old healthy single female patient presents with a twenty-four-hour history of right lower abdominal pain associated with vomiting six times and denied any history of fever, and she feels hungry. Exam revealed normal vital signs with mild right lower quadrant (RLQ) tenderness without rebound. Work up was normal. Which finding is against the diagnosis of appendicitis?

    A. Repeated vomiting
    B. Absence of fever
    C. Normal white blood cell count
    D. Presence of hunger

10. A 20-year-old male patient is admitted to the hospital with acute RLQ abdominal pain. Examination reveals tenderness and guarding in RLQ. Patient was taken to the OR. On table and after induction and intubation, you palpated the abdomen and felt a mass in RLQ. What is the best next action?

    A. Postpone surgery and wake the patient up

    B. Proceed with open appendectomy

    C. Proceed with laparoscopic exploration and appendectomy

    D. Convert to lower midline incision

Answer Key: 1 – D, 2 – B, 3 – C, 4 – A, 5 – C, 6 – B, 7 – D, 8 – A, 9 – D, 10 – A

COLORECTUM AND ANUS

1. **What would be the most appropriate bowel preparation regimen that can reduce risk of surgical site infection for a 62-year-old male patient undergoing low anterior resection for stage I rectal cancer?**

    A. Oral antibiotic
    B. Oral mechanical bowel preparation
    C. Rectal bowel preparation
    D. Chemical and mechanical bowel preparation

2. **A 50-year-old male patient is a known case of long-standing ulcerative colitis. Which of the following is an indication for total proctocolectomy?**

    A. Sclerosing cholangitis
    B. Aggressive polyarthritis
    C. Iron-deficiency anemia
    D. Refractory colitis

3. **A 50-year-old male patient is admitted to ICU for septic shock secondary to intrabdominal cause. He has history of abdominal pain and diarrhea with recent history of antibiotic use for pneumonia two weeks ago. What is the test of choice to diagnose C. difficile colitis**

    A. PCR for toxin gene
    B. Stool assay
    C. CT abdomen with oral and IV contrast
    D. Sigmoidoscopy to visualize pseudomembranes

4. **A 58-year-old male patient is a known case of long-standing ulcerative colitis. During screening colonoscopy, random biopsies were taken from the rectum. Pathology report showed sever dysplasia. What would be the best next option?**

    A. Repeat coloscopy in three months
    B. Confirm diagnosis by a second pathologist
    C. Colectomy with ileorectal anastomosis and mucosectomy
    D. Proctocolectomy

5. **A 51-year-old female patient two years post colectomy and ileorectal anastomosis for ulcerative colitis. Her follow-up proctoscopy and biopsy revealed mucosal inflammation with ulceration but no mass. What is the management option of choice?**

    A. CT abdomen with oral, IV, and rectal contrast
    B. PET/CT scan to rule out systemic disease
    C. Ciprofloxacin and metronidazole
    D. Resection of the remaining rectum with end ileostomy

6. **A 55-year-old male patient, known case of ulcerative colitis for twelve years, presents with severe, diffuse abdominal pain. Initial assessment showed temperature of 39°C, pulse of 113, BP of 100/68 with diffuse distention of the abdomen and mild tenderness. The X-ray abdomen showed right colon diameter of 16 cm. What is the initial management option of choice?**

    A. Decompressive colonoscopy urgently
    B. IV fluid and antibiotic with close monitoring
    C. Decompressive cecostomy
    D. Emergent subtotal collection and ileostomy

7. 66-year-old male patient three months post right hemi-colectomy for stage III colon cancer. He started the chemotherapy two weeks ago after which he presents with multiple mouth small ulceration and right lower quadrant pain. Vital signs are normal apart from tachycardia. Initial investigation revealed absolute neutrophil count of 450 cells/mm3 and thickened small bowel on abdominal radiography. Which of the following is CONTRINDICATED?

   A. CT angiogram
   B. Granulocyte-colony stimulation factors (G-CSF)
   C. Avoid antidiarrhea and narcotics
   D. Diagnostic colonoscopy

8. A 78-year-old male patient is brought to the ER with a twelve-hour history of constant central abdominal pain with nausea and vomiting. He is a case of paroxysmal atrial fibrillation. Examination reveals a distended abdomen with tenderness and guarding in the umbilical area and diminished bowel sounds. WBC is 24,000/mL. What is the most appropriate initial investigation?

   A. Abdominal X-ray
   B. CT scan with IV contrast to assess mesenteric vessels
   C. Sigmoidoscopy
   D. Conventional angiogram

9. **During abdominal exploration for suspecting mesenteric ischemia in a 77-year-old male patient, a pale 40-cm segment of jejunum was identified. What is the best next step?**

   A. Resection and primary anastomosis

   B. Resection and plan for second look

   C. Apply warm saline and increase FiO2 to 100% for 10 min and then reassess

   D. On-table conventional angiogram to confirm patency of mesenteric vessels with possible embolectomy

10. **A 68-year-old male patient is admitted to the hospital after he passed three large bloody stools. He passed moderate amount of blood with clots on arrival to ER. He is stable. Nasogastric aspirate is bilious. After fluid administration and laboratory. Which of the following is the most appropriate initial test in management?**

    A. Nuclear-tagged RBC scan

    B. CT angiogram

    C. Angiogram with selective embolization

    D. Colonoscopy

11. **A 55-year-old male patient presents with left lower abdominal pain of two-day duration, associated with constipation. On physical examination, he is febrile and has tenderness localized to the LLQ with fullness in that area. WBC is 22,000. What is the appropriate next step in management?**

    A. CT abdomen with PO and IV contrast

    B. Urgent colonoscopy

    C. Laparoscopic exploration

    D. Immediate laparotomy and resection with colostomy

12. **A 74-year-old female patient is a known case of recurrent attacks of uncomplicated sigmoid diverticulitis. She has history of hysterectomy for large fibroid. She presents with recurrent vaginitis. What would be the best tool to reach the diagnosis?**

    A. Rectal and genital examination
    B. Vaginogram
    C. CT abdomen/pelvis with barium enema
    D. Colposcopy and sigmoidoscopy

13. **A 38-year-old male patient presents to ER with symptoms and signs of sigmoid diverticulitis. He has mild tenderness and localized guarding in left side of the abdomen. Initial investigation showed leukocytosis, and CT abdomen suggests stage II by Hinchey classification with abscess size 5 × 5 cm adjacent to sigmoid colon. What is the best treatment option?**

    A. IV fluid and antibiotics and
    B. Transrectal drainage
    C. CT-guided percutaneous drainage
    D. Laparoscopic exploration with wide drainage

14. **A 43-year-old male patient presents was admitted to the surgical floor with the diagnosis of recurrent uncomplicated sigmoid diverticulitis for the third time (Hinchey I) within one year. Colon cancer was ruled out by colonoscopy. What is the best treatment option after discharge?**

    A. Continue conservative therapy
    B. Laparoscopic resection and primary anastomosis
    C. Hartmann's procedure
    D. Open resection and primary anastomosis

15. **A 58-year-old male patient presented to the hospital with picture suggestive of large bowel obstruction. What would be the most likely cause?**

    A. Adhesion
    B. Diverticulitis
    C. Volvulus
    D. Cancer

16. **A 70-year-old bedridden patient was brought to the ER with painless abdominal distention for few days. Vital signs are stable, and abdominal exam showed tense, nontender tympanic distended abdomen. You suspect Ogilvie's syndrome. What would be the most appropriate next management step?**

    A. NG tube decompression and correction of electrolyte
    B. Rectal tube decompression
    C. Lower gastrointestinal enema with gastrografin
    D. Urgent colonoscopy

17. **A 60-year-old male patient presented to the ER complaining of abdominal distension with discomfort and obstipation for two days. On examination, his abdomen was diffusely distended, tympanic with mild tenderness and sluggish bowel sounds. On PR, the rectum was empty. Vital signs were stable. There was marked colonic dilatation on X-ray. Rigid sigmoidoscopy revealed gradual narrowing of the lumen at 20 cm with a normal mucosa. What is the most likely diagnosis?**

    A. Sigmoid colon adenocarcinoma
    B. Volvulus
    C. Ulcerative colitis with stenotic segment
    D. Acute diverticulitis with mural narrowing

18. **A 55-year-old male patient presenting with absolute constipation of five days duration. An urgent CT showed a large mass at the rectosigmoid junction with dilated loops of large bowel. The cecal diameter is 11 cm. What would be the best line of management?**

    A. Nasogastric tube (NGT) suction and IV fluid for at least 48 hours and then reassess

    B. Sigmoidoscopy and biopsy confirmation of cancer

    C. Colonoscopy and stenting then full work up

    D. Colectomy and primary anastomosis +/- stoma

19. **A 20-year-old lady presents to the ER with persistent bloody diarrhea, abdominal cramps, and fever. Stool studies are negative for infectious cause. Colonoscopy reveals friable mucosa in a continuous manner from rectum to sigmoid. No granulomas are found on biopsy. Which of the following feature represent the most likely diagnosis?**

    A. Perianal fistula is a likely finding in MRI pelvis

    B. Pseudopolyp and cobblestones are common colonoscopy findings

    C. Rectal involvement is seen in colonoscopy

    D. Gastric involvement on gastroscopy is a common long-term complication

20. **A 52-year-old male patient is found to be anemic. Abdominal examination showed no organomegaly. but rectal examination and proctoscopy showed second-degree hemorrhoids. Based on these findings, what would be the next most appropriate management?**

    A. Stool occult blood test

    B. Barium enema

    C. CT abdomen with oral, IV, and rectal contrast

    D. Colonoscopy

21. **A 78-year-old male patient with history of ischemic heart disease developed abdominal pain. He looks dehydrated, but vital signs are ok. Mesenteric vascular occlusion is suspected. Which of the following is suggestive of this diagnosis?**

    A. Severe abdominal pain, more postprandial

    B. Vomiting of feculent material with streaks of blood

    C. Continuous bloody diarrhea with mucus

    D. Generalized severe tenderness with rebound and no bowel sound

22. **A colonic specimen was presented to the histopathologist following a large bowel resection. Which one of the following features is the most suggestive of ulcerative colitis?**

    A. Caseating necrosis

    B. Crypt abscess

    C. Multiple lymph node involvement

    D. Transmural thickening with granulomata and mucosal fibrosis

23. **A 25-year-old male patient presents to gastroenterology clinic with crampy abdominal pain and intermittent bloody diarrhea. Other review of system and abdominal/digital rectal exam are unremarkable. Sigmoidoscopy showed only hyperemia of rectal mucosa. Histopathology of rectal mucosa biopsy showed cryptitis with pseudopolyps. What would be your first line of therapy?**

    A. Sulfasalazine

    B. Oral prednisolone

    C. IV steroid

    D. Azathioprine or/and 6-MP (Mercaptopurine)

24. A 54-year-old female patient presents to ER with severe abdominal pain for few hours. She was recently diagnosed with acute myeloid leukemia and received the first session of chemotherapy. Her temperature is 36.5°C, and blood pressure is 98/59 with a pulse of 110. Her abdomen was distended and tender allover, mainly in the right lower quadrant. Initial blood test showed leukopenia with absolute neutrophil count of 450 cells/mm3. What would be the best treatment?

    A. Correct coagulopathy and avoid antidiarrhea/narcotics

    B. Resuscitation and broad-spectrum antibiotic

    C. Granulocyte-colony stimulation factors (G-CSF)

    D. Emergent total colectomy and ileostomy

25. A 77-year-old female patient presents to ER with painful swelling in the anal area with mild bleeding. She has diabetes, dyslipidemia, and ischemic cardiomyopathy. On rectal examination, there is an irreducible bluish/blackish protrusion through her anus with preserved grove between rectum and anus and visible circumferential mucosal folds. What would be the best treatment option?

    A. Conservative therapy with IV fluid and antibiotics

    B. Urgent hemorrhoidectomy

    C. Transabdominal rectal resection with rectopexy

    D. Perineal rectosigmoidectomy

26. **A 48-year-old female patient presents to surgery clinic with mild bleeding per rectum with the feel of fullness in the pelvic area. On rectal examination (digital and anoscope), there is first-degree uncomplicated hemorrhoid. Colonoscopy showed a rectal ulcer. Superficial biopsies were taken, which showed thickened mucosal layer and muscularis mucosa with distorted crypts. What would be the best next option?**

    A. Repeat colonoscopy for jumbo biopsies

    B. Defecography

    C. Dynamic pelvic MRI

    D. CT chest, abdomen, and pelvis to visceral spread

27. **A 65-year-old healthy male patient underwent screening colonoscopy that showed a sigmoid sessile polyp. Piecemeal biopsies were taken. The histopathology came back as invasive cancer with lymphovascular invasion. What would be the best treatment option?**

    A. Repeat colonoscopy in three months

    B. Repeat colonoscopy with complete mucosal resection

    C. Colotomy and competition polypectomy

    D. Formal cancer resection

28. A 56-year-old healthy male patient underwent screening colonoscopy that showed a sigmoid polyp. Polypectomy by hot snaring was performed. Twenty-four hours later, he presents to ER with left lower abdominal pain and fever. On examination, he is febrile with normal vitals and has localized tenderness in the let lower quadrant. Initial investigation revealed leukocytosis, and the chest X-ray was normal. What would be the best next step in management?

   A. Urgent 2-views abdominal X-ray
   B. Fluoroscopy with barium enema
   C. CT abdomen and pelvis
   D. Laparoscopic exploration with possible resection and/or diversion

29. A 16-year-old healthy female patient presents to the clinic because three of her family members (one of them is first degree) were diagnosed as hereditary non-polyposis colorectal cancer with positive mismatch repair gene (MMR) in the family. What is the first step in management?

   A. Genetic testing of the patient for MMR
   B. Screening colonoscopy
   C. Pelvic US to rule out associated ovarian cancer
   D. Prophylactic colectomy

30. **A 61-year-old healthy male patient underwent laparoscopic right hemicolectomy for invasive cancer. Histopathology showed complete resection with a clear margin of 5 mm with nine lymph nodes free of cancer. What would be your next step in management?**

    A. Close monitoring (clinical assessment, imaging, and colonoscopy)

    B. Discuss it in the multidiscipline tumor board

    C. Advice to go for chemo-radiotherapy

    D. Should perform re-resection

31. **A 63-year-old male patient one year post open left hemicolectomy and finished chemotherapy for stage III sigmoid cancer. During follow-up, he is asymptomatic, but the CEA is 9 ng/mL (normal 0–5 ng/mL) with normal labs, CT, and colonoscopy. What is the best next option?**

    A. Advice for cessation of smoking and reassess

    B. Follow-up in six months with clinical, laboratory, and imaging

    C. Positron emission tomography (PET) scan

    D. Exploration (laparotomy/laparoscopy) to rule out asymptomatic recurrence

32. **A 49-year-old female patient is following with colorectal cancer for investigation. What would be the best test to assess T1 tumor?**

    A. CT abdomen/pelvis with IV and rectal contrast

    B. Positron emission tomography (PET) scan

    C. MRI pelvis

    D. Endorectal ultrasound (ERUS)

33. A 39-year-old female patient presents to the ER with severe generalized abdominal pain, following a six-day history of obstipation. On exam, heart rate is 110 beats/minute, and blood pressure is 98/60. The abdomen is distended and rigid. Abdominal X-ray reveals large bowel obstruction. During laparotomy, there is a perforated, obstructed sigmoid neoplasm with fecal contamination. What is the best operative option?

   A. Resection and primary anastomosis
   B. Sigmoid resection and end colostomy
   C. Double-barrel colostomy
   D. Resection and plan for second procedure for anastomosis

34. A 45-year-old female patient is diagnosed 2-cm tumor mobile in rectal exam about 8 cm from anal verge. Work up, including ERUS, reveled a T1-localized tumor with no lymphovascular invasion. What is best next option?

   A. Low anterior resection
   B. Transanal excision (TAE)
   C. Transanal endoscopic surgery (TES)
   D. Neoadjuvant therapy and then restaging

35. A young male patient presents with anal discharge and itchiness. An anterior perianal opening with an internal opening below the dentate line were noted during exam. What is the best treatment option?

   A. Botox injection into the intersphincteric area
   B. Insertion of cutting seton and regular clinic visit to pull on the seton
   C. Fistulectomy and lateral sphincterotomy
   D. Fistulotomy

36. **A 31-year-old male patient presents to the surgical clinic with painless intermittent passage of bright red blood per rectum for several weeks. After history and physical examination, what is the next most appropriate initial step?**

    A. Anoscope
    B. Rigid proctosigmoidoscopy
    C. Flexible sigmoidoscopy
    D. Colonoscopy

37. **A 48-year-old heavy labor worker presented with bleeding per rectum. Proctoscopy revealed second-degree hemorrhoid with no evidence of active bleeding. What is the best treatment option?**

    A. Laser treatment
    B. Rubber banding
    C. Stapler hemorrhoidectomy
    D. Total hemorrhoidectomy

38. **A young female patient with Crohn's disease with anterior perianal fistula draining into the anal canal above the dentate line creating a trans-sphincteric type. What is the best treatment option?**

    A. Insertion of seton
    B. Biomedical plug and glue
    C. Fistulotomy
    D. Diverting colostomy

39. A 28-year-old female patient presents to clinic complaining of severe anal pain on defecation for two days following episode of constipation. There's no other significant medical history. Digital rectal examination was abandoned because of severe pain. What would be your initial management?

    A. Typical presentation of perianal spasm, reassure the patient, and prescribe analgesia and biofeedback exercise

    B. Dietary modification and calcium channel block local cream

    C. Prepare for examination under anesthesia

    D. Urgent lateral internal sphincterotomy

40. A 25-year-old patient presents with long-standing recurrent perianal pain and discharge. Local examination (lithotomy position) shows a small opening in relation to the anal ring at 8 o'clock. Where should be the internal opening located?

    A. 12 o'clock

    B. 3 o'clock

    C. 6 o'clock

    D. 9 o'clock

41. An 18-year-old male patient presents to the ER complaining of painful mass protruding out of his anus for the past four hours. He gave history of chronic constipation. On examination, there is a large, bluish mass protruding through his anus with ulceration but no active bleeding. What would be the most appropriate treatment?

    A. Transanal mucosal resection with anastomosis

    B. Incision and evacuation of hematoma

    C. Reduction under conscious sedation

    D. Cold compression, laxative, and analgesia

42. A 65-year-old female patient presents to the clinic with severe pruritis in Ano that failed all medical therapy. She underwent examination under anesthesia, and biopsy was taken from and 0.8 cm anal lesion. Histopathology came back as high grade anal intraepithelial neoplasia. What is the best next option?

    A. Observation every 12 months

    B. Wide local excision with topical 5-Fluorouracil

    C. Nigro protocol for 2 cycles, then reassessment

    D. Abdominoperineal resection (APR)

Answer Key: 1 – D, 2 – D, 3 – A, 4 – B, 5 – C, 6 – B, 7 – D, 8 – A, 9 – C, 10 – D, 11 – A, 12 – B, 13 – C, 14 – B, 15 – D, 16 – A, 17 – B, 18 – D, 19 – C, 20 – D, 21 – A, 22 – B, 23 – A, 24 – B, 25 – D, 26 – A, 27 – D, 28 – C, 29 – A, 30 – B, 31 – C, 32 – D, 33 – B, 34 – A, 35 – D, 36 – A, 37 – B, 38 – A, 39 – B, 40 – C, 41 – D, 42 – B

GASTROINTESTINAL BLEED

1. **A 59-year-old lady who's on diclofenac for osteoarthritis came to the ER with a one-day history of hematemesis and melena. Her hemoglobin level was 9 g/dL. The bleeding was controlled on upper GI endoscopy. Which of the following is associated with the highest risk for recurrent bleeding from a peptic ulcer?**

    A. Visible vessel within the ulcer
    B. Presence of erythematous mucosa surrounding the ulcer
    C. Presence of blood clots in the stomach
    D. A black spot in the ulcer's base

2. **A 57-year-old male patient was intubated and admitted to the ICU in severe sepsis and coagulopathy for five days. On Day 6, he developed bloody aspirate in the nasogastric tube with melena. What would be the most likely diagnosis in this patient?**

    A. Ruptured esophageal varices
    B. Mallory–Weiss syndrome
    C. Stress ulceration
    D. Dieulafoy's lesions

3. **A 65-year-old lady developed acute hematemesis with melena. She was scoped and was found to have a large ulcer on the posterior wall of duodenum. What is the most likely involved vessel?**

    A. Right gastric artery
    B. Left gastric artery
    C. Right arching gastroepiploic artery
    D. Branch of common hepatic artery

4. **A 65-year-old female patient present with melena and hypotension, which is corrected with resuscitation and blood transfusion. Upper GI endoscopy was normal. What is the next step in investigation?**

    A. Tagged RBC scan
    B. Colonoscopy
    C. Endoscopic-introduced capsule study
    D. Conventional angiogram

5. **A 70-year-old female patient who is known to have tachyarrhythmia is brought to ER with a history of crampy lower abdominal pain accompanied with bloody diarrhea for the past two days. On examination, there is left-sided abdominal tenderness. What is the most likely diagnosis?**

    A. Mesenteric ischemia
    B. Acute diverticulitis
    C. Ulcerative colitis
    D. Pseudomembranous colitis

6. **A 42-year-old female patient presents with passage of a large amount of dark red blood mixed with stool and clots twice shortly before coming to the ER associated with dizziness. Her vital signs were normal except for tachycardia, and her examination is normal except for dark blood on anoscope. Fluid resuscitation was started. What is the next most appropriate step to localize bleeding source?**

    A. Nasogastric tube
    B. Enteroscopy
    C. Octreotide scan
    D. CT angiogram of abdominal aorta and its branches

7. **A 65-year-old male patient, known case of aortic stenosis on treatment, presents with passage of a moderate amount of maroon colored stool four times over the past two days. Upper and lower GI endoscopies were unremarkable. What is the most likely cause?**

   A. Adenocarcinoma of the jejunum

   B. Arteriovenous malformation

   C. Aortoenteric fistula

   D. Crohn's disease of the ileum

8. **An 80-year-old male patient is brought to the ER with a twelve-hour history of constant central abdominal pain with nausea and vomiting. He has a history of atrial fibrillation on digoxin. Examination reveals a distended abdomen with mild tenderness but no rebound. WBC is 11,000/mL. CT angiogram confirmed the diagnosis of superior mesenteric artery thrombosis with enhanced small bowel. What is the best option?**

   A. Make him "Do Not Resuscitate – DNR" because of age and comorbidities

   B. Admit to ICU and start full anticoagulation and serial abdominal exam

   C. Angio-embolectomy +/- stenting

   D. Laparotomy, SMA embolectomy, and bowel resection

9. **A hemodynamically unstable 70-year-old male patient presents with a one-day history of bleeding per rectum. The amount of large. He is confused with a pulse rate of 138, blood pressure 98/60. Abdominal exam is unremarkable, and rectal exam and proctoscopy revealed fresh blood with clots. After stabilization, what would be the most appropriate step in management?**

   A. Resuscitation and close monitoring
   B. Colonoscopy
   C. Radionuclide imaging
   D. Selective angio-embolization

10. **A 48-year-old known case of uncontrolled Crohn's disease on medication presents to ER with bleeding per rectum. Proctoscopy revealed second-degree hemorrhoid with active bleeding. What is the best treatment option?**

   A. Suture ligation with packing
   B. Open hemorrhoidectomy
   C. Closed hemorrhoidectomy
   D. Stapler hemorrhoidectomy

Answer Key: 1 – A, 2 – C, 3 – D, 4 – B, 5 – A, 6 – A, 7 – B, 8 – C, 9 – D, 10 – A

SKIN, SOFT TISSUE, AND WOUND HEALING

1. **A 48-year-old male patient was discharged home after laparoscopic appendectomy for carcinoid tumor. How would you classify this wound?**

    A. Clean
    B. Clean-contaminated
    C. Contaminated
    D. Dirty

2. **A 58-year-old male patient presents with a mole on his forearm. What would be the feature suggestive of malignant melanoma?**

    A. Growing of hair out of the mole
    B. White discoloration
    C. Ulceration
    D. Diameter of 5 mm

3. **What would be the most effective method to avoid gas gangrene infection in a contaminated wound after a road car accident?**

    A. Anti-gas gangrene serum injection
    B. Closing the wound with nonabsorbable suture after wound wash
    C. Broad-spectrum IV antibiotic and regular wound check
    D. Wound irrigation and debridement

4. **A 70-year-old diabetic patient present to ER with a three-day history of painful right leg following a small puncture wound during gardening. She has temperature of 39°C, her leg is red, tender with bullae filled up with blood. What would be the most appropriate therapy in addition to antibiotics administration?**

    A. Immediate operative wide debridement
    B. Hyperbaric therapy
    C. Incision and drainage with packing and re-evaluation in 24 hours
    D. Urgent below knee amputation

5. **A 50-year-old female patient presents to ER with a well-demarcated, raised rapidly progressive red area in her left arm. She has chronic lymphedema of this arm following axillary dissection. What is the first line of antibiotic?**

    A. Penicillin G
    B. Ciprofloxacin
    C. Clindamycin
    D. Ceftriaxone

6. **The skin of mastectomy wound was closed with subcuticular 3/0 absorbable suture. What type of wound closure will take place?**

    A. Wound contraction
    B. Primary intention
    C. Secondary intention
    D. Tertiary intention

7. **A 23-year-old male patient presents to surgical clinic with discharging sinus in the intergluteal cleft. Which one of the following describes the best initial treatment for uncomplicated pilonidal sinus?**

    A. Incision and drainage
    B. Excision with primary closure
    C. Shaving and local hygiene
    D. Rhomboid flap is highly recommended

8. **A 44-year-old lady presents with a 1-cm left arm mole. What is the most appropriate method to confirm the diagnosis of melanoma?**

    A. Shaving biopsy
    B. Fine needle aspiration (FNA)
    C. Incisional biopsy
    D. Excisional biopsy

9. **A 44-year-old lady presents with a 1-cm left arm mole. What is the most appropriate method to confirm the diagnosis of melanoma?**

    A. Shaving biopsy
    B. Fine needle aspiration (FNA)
    C. Incisional biopsy
    D. Excisional biopsy

10. **A 38-year-old female patient underwent right hemicol-ectomy for large colonic polyp. On the sixth day, the patient starts complaining of pain inside the wound with serosanguinous fluid discharge from it. What is the most likely diagnosis?**

    A. Surgical site infection

    B. Wound dehiscence

    C. Anastomotic leak

    D. Necrotizing fasciitis

11. **A 52-year-old female patient with chronic burn nonheal-ing leg wound presented to the clinic with an ulcer over the medial malleolus. Her ankle–brachial Index (ABI) is 1.05. What is the likely type of ulcer?**

    A. Neuropathic

    B. Traumatic

    C. Venous

    D. Malignant

Answer Key: 1 – B, 2 – C, 3 – D, 4 – A, 5 – A, 6 – B, 7 – C, 8 – D, 9 – D, 10 – B, 11 – D

SURGICAL ENDOCRINOLOGY

1. **A 50-year-old female patient present with 1 × 1 cm thyroid nodule. Papillary thyroid cancer was confirmed by fine needle aspiration. What would be the most appropriate intervention?**

    A. Radioactive iodine ablation
    B. Lobectomy
    C. Lobectomy and isthmusectomy
    D. Total thyroidectomy

2. **A 30-year-old female patient presents for evaluation of a palpable thyroid nodule. Technetium-99m (99mTc) scan demonstrates a single cold nodule. The differential diagnosis includes which of the following?**

    A. Reidel thyroiditis
    B. Autoimmune nodule
    C. Neoplasm
    D. Autonomous nodule

3. **You have been called to see a 36-year-old male patient in the recovery room immediately after thyroid surgery; patient has developed sudden respiratory distress. The dressing was removed, and it was found to be slightly blood stained, and wound was bulging. What will be the first thing to be done?**

    A. Remove the stitch and then shift patient to OR
    B. Tracheostomy
    C. Cricothyroidotomy
    D. Laryngoscopy and intubation

4. **A biopsy from a rapidly enlarging thyroid gland in a patient with Hashimoto's thyroiditis. What is the most likely pathology you will find in the biopsy?**

    A. Thyroid lymphoma
    B. Papillary carcinoma
    C. Medullary carcinoma
    D. Anaplastic carcinoma

5. **Following total thyroidectomy, a 50-year-old female singer quit her job because she could not sing anymore. What would be the most likely cause?**

    A. Dense adhesion causing external compression on the larynx
    B. Injury to external laryngeal nerve
    C. Brachial plexus injury due to bad neck position during surgery
    D. Bilateral injury to the vocal cords

6. **The report of a fine-needle aspiration cytological (FNAC) examination from a solitary nodule in the left thyroid lobe of a patient indicates the presence of follicular neoplasm. What is the next most appropriate step in management?**

    A. Further investigation using I123 radio-isotope scan
    B. Reassurance and regular follow-up with repeated TSH, T3, and T4
    C. Repeated FNA
    D. Confirm the diagnosis by performing lobectomy

7. A 30-year-old female patient presents for evaluation of an enlarged thyroid gland. All the following are indications for surgery in this case EXCEPT.

    A. Severe exophthalmos
    B. Thyrotoxicosis
    C. Difficult breathing
    D. Suspicion of malignancy

8. A 25-year-old female patient presented with repeated attacks of watery nonoffensive diarrhea of a ten-day history of generalized fatigue and weakness. On examination, afebrile, pulse 102/minute, blood pressure 160/100, and the abdomen was free apart from exaggerated bowel sounds. Neck exam revealed diffusely enlarged, firm, nontender thyroid gland with palpable cervical chain of lymph nodes. What is the most likely cause?

    A. Sipple's syndrome
    B. Grave's disease
    C. Carcinoid syndrome
    D. Zollinger–Ellison syndrome

9. A 20-year-old female patient presents with an asymptomatic painless lump in the midline below her chin. The lump is smooth, measures 1 cm, is nontender, no discharge and moves on tongue protrusion. What would be the best treatment option?

    A. Antibiotic and observation
    B. Anti-thyroid medication
    C. Sistrunk procedure
    D. Thyroid lobectomy with isthmusectomy

10. The surgeon must be very careful while ligating arteries during thyroidectomy and not to injure the external laryngeal nerve. Which of the following artery runs close to this nerve?

    A. Superior thyroid artery
    B. Middle thyroid artery
    C. Inferior thyroid artery
    D. Thyroid ima

11. A patient underwent thyroid surgery. Post operatively, the patient is complaining of numbness and tingling around the mouth. What is the most likely diagnosis?

    A. Increased sodium retention
    B. Increased plasma volume
    C. Decreased plasma calcium
    D. Intra-operative nerve injury

12. A 59-year-old patient with a long history of chronic renal failure. During regular blood work, elevated calcium level was noted. What is the most likely etiology?

    A. Parathyroid carcinoma
    B. Parathyroid hyperplasia
    C. Parathyroid gland atrophy
    D. Functioning solitary parathyroid adenoma

13. A 56-year-old lady presented to the clinic with nipple discharge. Which one of the following suggests malignant cause?

    A. Greenish discharge
    B. Multiple ducts
    C. Spontaneous discharge
    D. Discharge from both nipples

14. **A 55-year-old lady underwent a left mastectomy and axillary dissection for breast cancer. After operation, she was found to have a winging scapula. She is otherwise well. What is the most likely cause?**

    A. Thoracodorsal nerve injury
    B. Long thoracic nerve injury
    C. Serratus anterior muscle injury
    D. Scapula dislocation

15. **A 59-year-old female patient presents to her family physician with a 3-cm palpable well-circumscribed, nontender breast mass that has increased in size. A subsequent mammogram shows no abnormalities. Which of the following is the next most appropriate step in the management?**

    A. Repeat mammogram in six months
    B. Tru-cut (core) biopsy for cytology
    C. Excisional biopsy
    D. Modified radical mastectomy

16. **A 40-year-old female patient is found to have a 2-cm, slightly tender cystic mass in her right breast. She has no palpable axillary lymph node. What would be the best course of action you will follow?**

    A. Reassurance and reexamination in the postmenstrual period
    B. Mammography and reevaluation of options with new information
    C. Immediate excisional biopsy
    D. Aspiration of the cyst for culture and cytologic analysis

17. **A 46-year-old mother of one child presented with small 1-cm mass of the left breast. Diagnosis of breast carcinoma in situ is highly suspected. What does carcinoma in situ mean?**

    A. Stage 1 breast cancer
    B. Cancer cells spread to areola-nipple complex
    C. Immature cancer cells
    D. Cancer cells do not cross basement membrane

18. **A 65-year-old female patient has clinical T2N0 estrogen receptor (ER)-positive breast cancer. Her breast is small in relation to tumor size. Which of the following is appropriate treatment plan?**

    A. Neoadjuvant therapy and then reassessment
    B. Lumpectomy, sentinel lymph node biopsy, and tamoxifen
    C. Lumpectomy, axillary dissection, and radiation
    D. Modified radical mastectomy

19. **A 70-year-old lady presents with few symptoms suggestive of breast cancer. Which one of the following is LEAST likely associated with inflammatory breast cancer?**

    A. Presence of breast mass
    B. Normal overlying skin
    C. Nipple inversion
    D. Axillary lymph node

20. **You have a patient in your clinic with breast cancer. She asked you about the meaning of sentinel lymph node (SLN). What will be your answer?**

    A. Any LN in the axilla tested positive in fine needle aspiration

    B. Normal overlying skin

    C. First LN that drains the breast cancer

    D. The positive LN after axillary LN dissection

21. **A 42-year-old female patient presents with 1 × 2 cm right breast painless mass for one month. Which of the following is NOT recommended step after taking detailed history and physical examination?**

    A. Breast ultrasound

    B. Mammogram

    C. Core needle biopsy

    D. Chest CT scan to rule out metastases

22. **A 21-year-old female patient presents to the clinic with a right breast lump few months following trauma to her right breast. Breast ultrasound raised the suspicion of cancer. What is the most likely diagnosis?**

    A. Ductal carcinoma in situ

    B. Radial scar

    C. Fat necrosis

    D. Duct ectasia

23. A 35-years-old female patient, who is currently breast-feeding her firstborn child, developed an erythematous and inflamed fluctuant area on breast examination. Which of the following steps in management is appropriate?

- A. Antibiotic to cover gram negative bacteria should be started
- B. Open drainage is likely indicated
- C. Stop breast feeding immediately and reassess the patient
- D. Biopsy should be considered regardless of the resolution of the pathology

24. A 21-year-old female patient presents with an asymptomatic breast mass. Which of the following would be an appropriate step in the management of this mass?

- A. Ultrasound is useful in the differential diagnosis
- B. Mammography will play a role in the diagnosis
- C. Core biopsy is the best method to confirm your suspicion
- D. Excision should be done to obtain final diagnosis

25. A 42-year-old female patient presents with 2 × 2 cm right breast painless mass for one month. Bilateral mammogram was done. Which one of the following mammographic features is suggestive of malignancy?

- A. Macrocalcification in mammogram
- B. Visible lymph node in the axilla
- C. Nodular breast tissue
- D. Loss of breast architecture

26. A 48-year-old female patient presents to the clinic with an ill-defined 2-cm mass in the outer upper quadrant of her right breast for six months. Which of the following would be the most appropriate step to give you the final diagnosis?

    A. Ultrasound-guided FNA
    B. Excisional biopsy
    C. Core biopsy
    D. Stereotactic biopsy

Answer Key: 1 – D, 2 – C, 3 – A, 4 – A, 5 – B, 6 – D, 7 – A, 8 – A, 9 – C, 10 – A, 11 – C, 12 – B, 13 – C, 14 – B, 15 – B, 16 – D, 17 – D, 18 – A, 19 – B, 20 – C, 21 – D, 22 – C, 23 – B, 24 – A, 25 – D, 26 – C

PRINCIPLES OF TRAUMA

1. A 26-year-old male patient was brought to the ER after a motor vehicle crash. You suspected severe head injury. What is the most important initial step in management of this patient?

    A. Avoid hypoxia
    B. Support the circulation
    C. Urgent CT brain
    D. Determine the GCS score

2. A 36-year-old female patient was ejected from the car during a head-on collision with a truck. On arrival to the ER, she is cold and clammy peripherally with decreased urine output. Her pulse rate is 120 beats/minute, and blood pressure is 80/60 mmHg. She has engorged neck veins. Her chest is clear with equal and good air entry on both sides on auscultation. What is the most likely diagnosis?

    A. Massive hemothorax
    B. Tension pneumothorax
    C. Cardiac tamponade
    D. Aortic rupture

3. A 29-year-old male patient was brought to ER after he fell from three stories. Primary survey was normal EXCEPT that he opens his eye to verbal stimuli, localize painful stimuli with his hand, and produce incomprehensive sound. What would be his Glasgow Coma Scale (GCS)?

    A. 4
    B. 6
    C. 8
    D. 10

4. **A 25-year-old male patient is brought to a hospital to be seen by a general surgeon after being involved in a motor vehicle crash. He was stable hemodynamically. Computed tomography shows an aortic injury and splenic laceration with free abdominal fluid. His blood pressure falls to 70/40 mm Hg after CT. What would be the most appropriate step in management?**

    A. Conventional angiography with stenting of the aortic injury
    B. Exploratory laparotomy
    C. Infuse more crystalloids intravenously
    D. Transfer to a higher-level trauma center

5. **A 28-year-old male patient was injured in a motorcycle accident in which he was not wearing a helmet. On admission to the ER, he was hypotensive with GCS of 7. He was bleeding profusely from the nose and had an obviously open femur fracture. Breath sounds were decreased on the right side of the chest. What is the first initial management?**

    A. Endotracheal intubation with in-line cervical traction
    B. Obtain intravenous access and begin emergency type O blood transfusions
    C. Tube thoracostomy in the right hemithorax
    D. Control of hemorrhage with anterior and posterior nasal packing

6. **A 20-year-old male patient was involved in a fight. He is complaining of left upper quadrant pain. His heart rate is 90 beats/minute, and his blood pressure is 110/71 mmHg. He has localized tenderness in the left upper quadrant. His hemoglobin is within normal range. Abdominal CT scan showed grade II splenic injury. What would be the appropriate management?**

    A. Bed rest and close observation in the intensive care unit
    B. Abdominal angiogram to see whether there is bleeding
    C. Laparotomy and repair of the spleen
    D. Laparotomy and splenectomy

7. **A 26-year-old female patient was ejected from the car during a head-on collision with a truck. On arrival to the ER, she has stable vital signs and left upper quadrant tenderness without signs of peritonitis. What is the most appropriate next step in the management of the abdominal pain?**

    A. Admission for observation and serial abdominal exam
    B. Diagnostic peritoneal lavage (DPL)
    C. Focused assessed of sonography for trauma (FAST)
    D. Exploratory laparotomy

8. A 42-year-old female patient complains of left upper
    abdominal pain worse on respiration and radiate to
    the left scapula on Day 7 post splenectomy after motor
    vehicle crash. Examination reveals a temperature of
    38.6°C, decreased air entry on the left side, and left upper
    quadrant abdominal tenderness. What is the most likely
    postsplenectomy complication?

    A. Basal atelectasis
    B. Gastric perforation
    C. Portal vein thrombosis
    D. Subphrenic abscess

9. A 21-year-old patient was involved in a motorcycle
    crash. He was brought to emergency department by Red
    Crescent ambulance. Your supervisor said, "This patient is
    in class II shock." On which of the following did he base
    his impression?

    A. Tachycardia
    B. Hypotension
    C. Reduced level of consciousness
    D. Reduced urine output

10. **A 45-year-old male patient, involved in motor vehicle crash, presented to ER complaining of severe right chest pain. Airway is intact. On breathing, he has diminished right chest expansion with paradoxical movement with crepitation on palpation and reduced air entry on auscultation. O2 saturation is 93% on room air. Pulse is 109, and blood pressure is 160/98. He is in severe pain. Chest X-ray showed three fractured ribs in more than two places. What is the best treatment option?**

   A. Prophylactic intubation should be performed

   B. Pain control, pulmonary toilet, and supplemental oxygen

   C. Fluid restriction and diuresis are indicated

   D. Immediate transfer to operating room for rib fixation

11. **A 21-year-old male patient, involved in motorcycle crash, presented to ER with GCS of 7 with bruised both eyes, tachycardic, and hypotensive. Anesthesia doctor is about to perform rapid sequence intubation. Which of the following induction agents is appropriate?**

   A. Thiopental

   B. Ketamine

   C. Propofol

   D. Etomidate

12. **An 18-year-old male patient, involved in motorcycle crash, presented to ER with GCS of 11 in class III shock. Which of the following is a poor prognostic factor?**

   A. Alkalosis

   B. Scoring of motor component of GCS is 6

   C. Hyperchloremia

   D. Hyperthermia

13. A 22-year-old male patient, involved in a fight, presented to ER intoxicated and is in class III shock. During initial assessment and resuscitation, blood pressure had transient response to fluid challenge, and abdomen is distended but difficult to assess due to mental status. DPL was performed for equivocal FAST. DPL showed RBC 80,000 RBC/mm3, WBC 700 WBC/mm3, and amylase 200 IU. What is the next step?

    A. Admit for observation and serial abdominal exam

    B. CT abdomen to rule out intraabdominal

    C. Diagnostic laparoscopy

    D. Exploratory laparotomy

14. A 35-year-old male patient was brought by the EMS after he fell from three stories. After assessment and resuscitation, he sustained isolated severe (GSC 7) head injury with CT head positive for subdural hematoma with midline shift. What is the best treatment option after intubation and resuscitation?

    A. Craniotomy

    B. Intracranial pressure monitoring with drainage

    C. Deep sedation and paralysis

    D. Mannitol, anticonvulsant, and repeat CT brain in twenty-four hours

15. A 17-year-old male patient presents to ER with epistaxis following a fight. He is full conscious and able to talk freely. Initial assessment revealed nasal fracture with bleeding. What is the best initial option to stop bleeding?

    A. Urgent OR for nasal reduction and bleeding control

    B. Angio-embolization of the ethmoid vessels

    C. Direct pinching of the nose

    D. Bilateral nasal packing

16. **A 30-year-old female patient was brought to Level 1 trauma center after she sustained a gunshot to the neck. During initial assessment, the patient is awake and communicating well and is hemodynamically stable. Local examination showed entry wound on the left side of the neck above the level of cricoid cartilage with expanding hematoma. What is the best initial step in management?**

    A. Endotracheal intubation
    B. Cricothyroidotomy
    C. Urgent CT neck with IV contrast to rule out major vascular injury
    D. Local wound exploration in ER and packing

17. **A 21-year-old male patient presents to the ER after he was stabbed to the right neck during a fight. He is drowsy and mumbling. Heart is 110 with SBP 95. The single wound is located on the right side just above sternal notch. The patient was intubated and resuscitated, but blood pressure is not stabilizing. What would be the best treatment option?**

    A. Angio-embolization
    B. Anterior neck exploration
    C. Right high-level thoracotomy with trap door incision
    D. Sternotomy with possible clavicular extension

18. **During anterior neck exploration for stab wound through an oblique incision along the anterior border of sternomastoid muscle, what structure will the surgeon encounter that is called neck gatekeeper?**

    A. Carotid sheath
    B. Facial vein
    C. Hypoglossal nerve
    D. Omohyoid muscle

19. **A 19-year-old male patient presents to ER after motor vehicle crash. He is disoriented and complaining of severe right chest pain. During primary survey, his O2 saturation is 88% on room air and no breath sound on the left subcutaneous emphysema. Heart rate is 120 beats/minute but blood pressure in 80/60. What is optimum next action?**

    A. Intubation

    B. Chest tube insertion

    C. Needle decompression

    D. Video-assisted thoracoscopy

20. **A 40-year-old female patient presents to ER after she was hit by a car when she was crossing the road. She is not responding to painful stimuli. Which one of the following assessment tools is used during primary survey to rule out thoracic injury?**

    A. Extended focused assessment of sonography for trauma (eFAST)

    B. CT scan of the chest with IV contrast

    C. Awake bronchoscopy

    D. Conventional aortogram to rule out life-threating vascular injury

21. **A 58-year-old male patient, a known case of bronchial asthma, presents to ER with severe chest blunt trauma after a fight. He has four left-sided rib fractures at two sites along each rib with paradoxical chest wall movement. He is in severe pain, stable blood pressure, pulse of 110 beats/minute with O2 saturation of 89% on 4L nasal cannula. What is the most likely cause of his desaturation?**

    A. Flail chest

    B. Tracheal injury

    C. Stress (trauma)-induced asthma exacerbation

    D. Lung contusion

22. **A 59-year-old female patient was brought to ER after she fell downstairs. Initial assessment revealed only SaO2 88% on RA. She sustained two rib fractures on the right side with moderate pulmonary contusion. No other injuries were identified. What would be the LEAST appropriate treatment option?**

    A. Fluid restriction

    B. Intravenous steroid to reduce risk of ARDS

    C. High O2 flow nasal cannula

    D. Invasive ventilation

23. **A 38-year-old male patient was involved in a fight. He came to ER complaining of SOB and left chest pain. Initial assessment/imaging revealed left flail chest with moderate pulmonary contusion. Pan scan showed flail chest with severe rib displacement. What is the best pain management plan?**

    A. Patient control analgesia (PCA) using morphine

    B. Intrapleural/intercostal infusion of fentanyl

    C. Epidural analgesia

    D. Rib fixation

24. **A 48-year-old male patient was admitted for observation after he fell down the stairs. All his assessments were normal including CXR. CT chest showed a small rim of hemopneumothorax. Which one of the following has the weakest evidence in reducing empyema risk?**

    A. Aseptic technique during chest tube insertion

    B. Drain all hemopneumothoraxes

    C. Prophylactic antibiotic

    D. Inserting the chest tube in the OR

25. A 52-year-old female patient was admitted for observation after she was involved in car accident (front passenger, belted). All her assessments were normal including CXR. CT chest showed an aortic intimal injury with small flap. What is the best treatment option?

    A. Anti-hypertensive medication and antiplatelet

    B. Anticoagulation

    C. Endovascular stenting

    D. Sternotomy and aortic repair with possible use of graft

26. A 23-year-old male patient was admitted after he was involved in car (T-boned) accident as a driver. All his assessments were normal except CXR, which showed elevation of the left diaphragm. How would you confirm the presence of diaphragmatic injury?

    A. Clinically and chest radiography

    B. Chest CT scan with oral and IV contrast

    C. MRI chest

    D. Laparoscopy

27. A 43-year-old female patient was hit by a car when she was crossing the street. She is stable with GCS 12. After assessment, pan CT revealed small subdural hematoma, grade V liver injury with no blush and moderate-to large hemoperitoneum with no pneumoperitoneum. What would be the appropriate treatment?

    A. Close monitoring in the ICU

    B. Angiogram with/without embolization

    C. Diagnostic laparoscopy to rule out associated injuries

    D. Emergency laparotomy

28. **A 37-year-old male patient was brought to ER one hour after MVC. Airway and breathing were Ok. He is complaining of RUQ pain. He is stable but has generalized tenderness with positive FAST. What would be an appropriate management?**

   A. Resuscitate and then take him to CT for whole body imaging

   B. Start tranexamic acid and reassess

   C. Take him to angiogram for embolization

   D. For OR immediately

29. **A 33-year-old female patient was hit by a car when she was crossing the street. She is stable with GCS 13. After resuscitation, pan CT revealed grave IV liver injury with NO blush and minimal hemoperitoneum. Patient was admitted for close monitoring. On Day 5 in the ICU, she started having abdominal distention and difficulty in breathing with tachycardia and fever. No changes in blood pressure or hemoglobin. Abdomen is distended, tender, and positive for ascites. What would be your next step after resuscitation?**

   A. Emergent laparotomy

   B. Bed-side US and tapping

   C. CT abdomen and pelvic with IV and oral contrast

   D. Urgent magnetic resonance cholangiopancreatography (MRCP)

30. **During exploratory laparotomy for a trauma patient who presented with peritonitis following a fight, you found a small tear in small bowel mesentery which was sutured. During exploration, grade III pancreatic injury in the tail was identified. What is the most appropriate action?**

    A. Finish exploration and leave it alone
    B. Intraoperative pancreatography and if there is ductal injury perform distal pancreatectomy
    C. Wide local drainage
    D. Spleen-preserving distal pancreatectomy and drain insertion

31. **A 17-year-old boy presents to the ER with abdominal pain after he hit his abdomen against bicycle handle. He was stable with localized tenderness on the epigastrium. CT showed laceration in the body of the pancreas. What would be the best approach?**

    A. Admit for observation
    B. MRCP/ERCP
    C. Diagnostic laparoscopy
    D. Exploratory laparotomy

32. **A 50-year-old female patient came to the ER after she got shot in her abdomen. She is conscious with stable hemodynamic. Exam revealed an entry wound in the right upper quadrant and exist wound in the right flank. Her abdomen is tender just around wounds. Rest of primary and secondary survey are normal. What is the best next option in the management?**

    A. Admit for close monitoring and serial exam
    B. Local wound exploration
    C. CT abdomen
    D. Diagnostic laparoscopy

33. A 30-year-old female patient came to the ER after she got stabbed in her abdomen. She is conscious and stable hemodynamic. Examination revealed stab wound in left lower quadrant. There is no evisceration and bleeding. Her abdomen is tender just around the wound. Rest of primary and secondary survey are normal. What is the best next step?

   A. Discharge home after twenty-four hours monitoring
   B. FAST, admit for observation if negative
   C. CT abdomen with triple (IV, oral and rectal) contrast
   D. Local wound exploration

34. An 18-year-old male patient presented to ER with rectal bleeding after he fell on a wood stick. He is stable but complaining of lower abdominal pain. CT abdomen showed minimal abdominal fluid and no pneumoperitoneum. What is the next step in management?

   A. Conservative therapy with NPO and IV antibiotic
   B. Barium rectal contrast
   C. Pelvic magnetic resonance imaging (MRI)
   D. Proctosigmoidoscopy

35. A 29-year-old male patient was brought to ER after he got stabbed with a knife just below the left nipple. He is confused and in shock with muffled heart sound. Fluid resuscitation has started. What would be the most important next option?

   A. Three-way adhesive dressing
   B. Needle decompression followed by chest tube if positive
   C. DPL followed by laparotomy if positive
   D. Pericardial window

36. **A 29-year-old male patient was picked up by the EMS following bad car crash. Which of the following given in the prehospital period could improve outcome for patients suspecting hemorrhagic shock?**

    A. Recombinant factor VII
    B. Vitamin K
    C. Tranexamic acid
    D. Tourniquet applied to the crushed limb

37. **Paramedics are on the way to respond to a call from a patient who was involved in a major fight. When they arrived, they found him unconscious and shocked. Major abdominothoracic and head injuries are suspected. Which of the following should be done in the ambulance and shown to improve outcome?**

    A. Administer 2 L of crystalloid
    B. Start plasma transfusion
    C. 500 mL of colloid administration
    D. 100 mL of 3% saline to minimize brain edema

38. **A 45-year-old male patient sustained a gunshot wound (GSW) to the abdomen with unclear time of injury. He arrived in ED and got intubated for GCS 5. Initial assessment revealed severe hemorrhagic shock with entry wound in the RUQ with distended abdomen. Which of the following is proven to improve outcome?**

    A. Initiation of massive transfusion protocol
    B. Fluid resuscitation to maintain palpable central pulses
    C. Thromboelastographic (TEG)-directed transfusion
    D. Administration of recombinant F VII

39. An unknow patient was found in the street unconscious and brought by EMS to ER intubated. Initial assessment revealed hemorrhagic shock with distended abdomen and possible open-book pelvic fracture. He is going to the OR, and massive transfusion protocol was initiated. Which ratio has been associated with better outcome?

    A. 1:1:2

    B. 2:1:1

    C. 1:1:1

    D. 1:2:1

40. Blood test was sent for major trauma patient with suspected massive retroperitoneal bleed from pelvic trauma. Which of the following marker is associated with increased mortality?

    A. Prolongation of prothrombin time (PT)

    B. Falling of fibrinogen level

    C. Thrombocytopenia

    D. Near normal level of hemoglobin

41. A 47-year-old male patient fell from the fourth floor and landed on concrete. Initial assessment revealed GCS of 10 and diminished breath sound bilaterally and hypotension. Initial imaging showed possible bilateral hemothorax, and the FAST was negative. What would be the most appropriate action?

    A. Resuscitate and send for pan CT scan once stable

    B. ICU admission for observation

    C. Official abdominal ultrasound then decides

    D. Perform diagnostic peritoneal lavage (DPL)

42. **A 30-year-old female patient was brought to ED by EMS after she fell from three stories. Initial assessment and resuscitation revealed Class III shock. Which of the following is accurate predictor of shock class?**

    A. Systolic blood pressure <100
    B. Hemoglobin and hematocrit
    C. Lactate level
    D. Base deficit

43. **A 40-year-old male patient was brought to ED by EMS after he was hit by a car. Initial assessment and resuscitation revealed hypovolemic shock. Which of the following predict transfusion requirement?**

    A. Central venous pressure
    B. Initial hemoglobin and hematocrit
    C. Base deficit
    D. Size of the fluid collection in Morison's pouch on FAST

44. **A 17-year-old female patient was taken to the OR after a bad motor vehicle crash (MVC). Intraoperative finding includes Grade III splenic injury, small and large bowel injuries. Patient is unstable and acidotic. Which of the following will improve outcome?**

    A. Splenorraphy, bowel resection, and anastomosis
    B. Splenorraphy and staple off all injured bowel ends
    C. Splenectomy and resection of injured bowel
    D. Just pack and take her to ICU for second look in forty-eight hours

45. A 25-year-old male patient was involved in roll-over MVC and ejection. He arrived intubated for low GCS. He responded to fluid challenge. There is obvious deformity of both femurs. What would be the best management option?

    A. Whole body CT scan

    B. FAST, X-ray, and then reassess

    C. X-ray, FAST, and then selective CT scan

    D. Selective CT scan

Answer Key: 1 – A, 2 – C, 3 – D, 4 – B, 5 – A, 6 – A, 7 – C, 8 – D, 9 – A, 10 – B, 11 – D, 12 – C, 13 – D, 14 – A, 15 – C, 16 – A, 17 – D, 18 – B, 19 – C, 20 – A, 21 – D, 22 – B, 23 – C, 24 – D, 25 – A, 26 – D, 27 – A, 28 – D, 29 – B, 30 – C, 31 – B, 32 – C, 33 – D, 34 – D, 35 – D, 36 – C, 37 – B, 38 – A, 39 – C, 40 – B, 41 – A, 42 – D, 43 – C, 44 – C, 45 – B

CRITICAL CARE

1. A 59-year-old male patient is brought to the ER in pro-
    found hypovolemic shock from massive hematemesis
    requiring resuscitation with 6 L of crystalloid solution and
    8 units of packed RBCs. The patient starts to bleed from
    IV-line site and in the urine. What is the most likely cause?

    A. Alkalosis
    B. Hypothermia
    C. Transfusion-related infectious complication
    D. Hypercalcemia

2. A 30-year-old male patient was admitted with acute
    cholecystitis and started on conservative treatment. After
    few hours, he developed sudden onset of severe short-
    ness of breath, no chest pain, and diffuse wheeze in the
    chest. His blood pressure was 70/30, and pulse rate was
    120 beats/minute. What is the most likely diagnosis?

    A. Acute pulmonary embolism
    B. Progressing into gangrenous gallbladder
    C. Anaphylactic shock
    D. Acute coronary syndrome

3. A trauma patient has been resuscitated for hypovolemic
    shock. Which one of the following is an ineffective fluid
    for expanding plasma volume?

    A. Normal saline
    B. Ringer lactate
    C. Albumin solution
    D. 5% dextrose in water

4. **A 31-year-old female patient was hit by a bus. She was brought to the ER for management. You suspected the presence of shock. Which of the following must be present to confirm your diagnosis?**

    A. Hypoxemia

    B. Acidosis

    C. Hypotension

    D. Evidence of inadequate organ perfusion

5. **A 67-year-old female patient is admitted to the ICU for managing COPD exacerbation with Bi-PAP. The patient is restless but conscious and cooperative. Which of the following is appropriate to give to calm her down?**

    A. Dexmedetomidine

    B. Fentanyl

    C. Midazolam

    D. Haloperidol

6. **A 76-year-old healthy male patient is admitted to cardiac unit with new onset rapid atrial fibrillation. He is dizzy with chest tightness. His blood pressure is 144/89. What is the treatment of choice?**

    A. Amiodarone 300 mg IV bolus over 10 min

    B. Metoprolol

    C. Digoxin

    D. Cardioversion

7. **A 76-year-old healthy male patient is admitted to cardiac unit with new onset rapid atrial fibrillation. He is asymptomatic with blood pressure of 144/89. You managed to slow the rate but after forty-eight hours with IV medication. What is appropriate to be done next?**

    A. Perform transesophageal echocardiogram
    B. Start IV heparin infusion
    C. Switch the medication to oral formula
    D. Percutaneous angiography and catheter ablation

8. **A 55-year-old male patient is admitted to the surgical floor post uneventful laparoscopic cholecystectomy for gallstone. He has a coronary stent placed one year ago, and he was on antiplatelet. Few hours later, he developed chest pain radiating to the left shoulder. What would be your immediate next step?**

    A. Give oxygen by nasal cannula
    B. Nitrate sublingual
    C. Morphine
    D. Aspirin 325 mg orally

9. **An 80-year-old male patient presents to the ER of a tertiary hospital with typical chest pain. Initial assessment revealed ST elevation myocadiac infarction. What would be the ideal perfusion therapy?**

    A. IV heparin infusion with a target partial thromboplastin time (PTT) between 50 and 70
    B. Give thrombolytics with door-to-injection three hours
    C. Percutaneous coronary intervention with door-to-balloon <90 min
    D. Coronary artery bypass graft (CABG)

10. **A 38-year-old male patient is admitted to ICU following severe traumatic brain injury. He is intubated and mechanically ventilated. Which of the following will increase the risk of ventilation-associated pneumonia?**

    A. Deep sedation without interruption

    B. Using mouth wash to keep good oral hygiene

    C. Elevation of the bed head to 45 degrees

    D. Use of endotracheal tube with subglottic port for suction

11. **A 22-year-old female patient is admitted to ICU as a case of septic shock for perforated appendix. She is on minimal mechanical ventilation setting. Which of the following with indicate extubation will likely be successful in this patient?**

    A. Patient is awake but agitated

    B. Rapid-shallow breathing index is 80

    C. Minute ventilation is >15 L/minute

    D. Absent cuff leak

12. **A 59-year-old female patient is admitted to ICU as case of hemorrhagic shock following assault. She came back from OR after splenectomy and massive transfusion. Her mechanical ventilation setting is FiO2 80% with PaO2 60 on arterial blood gas. Chest X-ray showed bilateral infiltrate. What is the most likely diagnosis?**

    A. Transfusion-related acute lung injury (TRALI)

    B. Severe negative-pressure pulmonary edema

    C. Severe lung contusion with aspiration

    D. Acute respiratory distress syndrome

13. **A 70-year-old male patient presents to the ER with generalized peritonitis. The diagnosis of septic shock from perforated gut is suspected. Which of the following will be abnormally elevated in relation to acid–base balance?**

   A. Lactate level
   B. Concentration of bicarbonate
   C. Blood pH
   D. Arterial PaCO2

14. **Four days after uneventful cholecystectomy, an asymptomatic middle-aged female patient is found to have a serum sodium level of 125 mEq/L. She has been in clear fluid diet and water during this period. Which of the following is appropriate initial management?**

   A. Administer hypertonic saline solution
   B. Restriction of free water
   C. Aggressive diuresis with lasix
   D. Oral replacement with sodium chloride tablet

15. **A trauma patient has been resuscitated for hypovolemic shock. Which one of the following is fluid for initial plasma expansion?**

   A. 10% albumin
   B. 0.9% normal saline
   C. Ringer lactate
   D. 3% hypertonic saline

16. **A 50-year-old homeless male patient was brought to the ER in a stuporous state. Blood pressure is 100/50 mmHg, heart rate 120 beats/minute, respiratory rate 35/minute, and temperature is 40°C. He was found to have cellulitis of his left foot. Below are his lab results: Sodium 150 mEq/L, Potassium 2.5 mEq/L, pH 7.2, PCO2 25 mmHg, and bicarbonate 10 mEq/L. What is the acid–base status?**

    A. Metabolic acidosis with partial respiratory compensation

    B. Metabolic acidosis

    C. Respiratory acidosis

    D. Respiratory alkalosis with complete metabolic compensation

17. **A 57-year-old male patient was intubated and admitted to the ICU in severe sepsis and coagulopathy two days after laparotomy for perforated appendix. On Day 5, he developed bloody aspirate in the nasogastric tube with melena. What is the likely diagnosis?**

    A. Ruptured esophageal varices

    B. Mallory–Weiss syndrome

    C. Dieulafoy's lesion

    D. Stress ulceration

18. **A 68-year-old male patient presented to ER with massive upper GI bleeding. Massive transfusion protocol was initiated. What would be the most likely complication associated with massive blood transfusion?**

    A. Hypokalemia

    B. Hypocalcemia

    C. Hyponatremia

    D. Hypophosphatemia

19. **A 76-year-old male patient is admitted to ICU in septic shock from infected stage IV bedsore. During initial assessment and resuscitation, which of the following has proven to improve outcome in this patient?**

    A. Invasive monitoring with pulmonary catheter to assess LV function
    B. Early administration of norepinephrine
    C. Intravenous antibiotics
    D. Early cortisone administration

20. **A 58-year-old female patient is admitted to ICU after a fall, for which she was intubated with low GCS. The diagnosis of ventilation-associated pneumonia on Day 4 post ICU admission is suspected. What would be the best way to confirm the diagnosis?**

    A. Chest X-ray to confirm the presence of infiltrate
    B. Elevation of inflammatory markers
    C. Sputum culture
    D. Tracheal aspiration

21. **An 80-year-old female patient is admitted to ICU as a case of aspiration pneumonia with multiorgan failure for which she got intubated and mechanically ventilated. Which of the following factors carries the highest risk for stress gastric ulcer?**

    A. Coagulopathy
    B. Age
    C. Sepsis
    D. Female gender

22. A 78-year-old female patient is admitted to the ICU as a case of infected stage IV bedsore with osteomyelitis for which she needed a six – to eight-week course of antibiotics. Which of the following will increase the risk of catheter-related blood stream infection?

    A. Use peripherally inserted central catheter

    B. Change peripheral line every five to six days

    C. Insertion of jugular line instead of femoral line

    D. IV team inserts and manages the central line

Answer Key: 1 – B, 2 – C, 3 – D, 4 – D, 5 – A, 6 – D, 7 – B, 8 – A, 9 – C, 10 – A, 11 – B, 12 – D, 13 – A, 14 – B, 15 – C, 16 – A, 17 – D, 18 – B, 19 – C, 20 – D, 21 – A, 22 – B

PEDIATRIC, VASCULAR, AND THORACIC SURGERIES

1. A seven-year-old boy is brought to the ER after he was hit by a car. He is in shock. What would be the ideal fluid resuscitation, keeping in mind that his body weight is 20 kilograms?

    A. 200 mL bolus
    B. 300 mL bolus
    C. 400 mL bolus
    D. 600 mL bolus

2. An 8-year-old boy presents to the clinic with painful central neck swelling. It has been there for few months and was moving with tongue protrusion, but lately, it became bigger, painful, red, and not mobile. It is associated with fever. Ultrasound of the neck showed feature suggestive of an abscess. What is the treatment of choice?

    A. Oral antibiotic and follow-up
    B. Aspiration under aseptic technique
    C. Incision and drainage
    D. Total excision

3. A 2-day-old baby girl was admitted with drooling, vomiting, regurgitation, and chocking causing mild respiratory distress but stable hemodynamically. Passing a nasogastric tube has failed. Chest X-ray revealed no gas in the stomach. Which of the following could be harmful in this patient?

    A. Insertion of NGT under guidance
    B. Start IV antibiotic
    C. Positive pressure ventilation
    D. Prepare the baby for early surgical intervention in one to two days

4. **A 3-week-old baby boy was brought by his mother (heavy smoker) to the ER for nonbilious projectile vomiting. Initial assessment revealed a palpable upper abdominal mass. Ultrasound showed a target sign. What is the best management option?**

    A. Endoscopic dilation
    B. Gastrojejunal bypass
    C. Distal gastrectomy with duodeno-gastric anastomosis
    D. Pyloromyotomy

5. **A 3-year-old boy was brought by his mother to the clinic because she noticed the boy is holding his head and crying. On exam, his blood pressure is elevated, and abdominal exam revealed a mass in right flank extending toward midline. What is the most likely diagnosis?**

    A. Neuroblastoma
    B. Wilms tumor
    C. Hepatocellular carcinoma
    D. Teratoma

6. **A 56-year-old male patient is admitted to ICU with right sided ischemic stroke, which was confirmed by CT scan. Initial work up showed 40% stenosis of right internal carotid artery with ulceration on MRA. What is the best treatment option?**

    A. Aspirin and clopidogrel
    B. Angiogram and stenting
    C. Carotid endarterectomy
    D. Resection of the affected segment and interposition graft insertion

7. **A 51-year-old male patient (known hypertensive and smoker) presents with lower sternal sharp pain radiating to the right side of the abdomen and associated with shortness of breath and sweating. He is tachycardic with systolic blood pressure is 98 with tenderness in the epigastrium. Initial workup showed ST depression in inferior leads with mild elevation of T-troponin. What is the best management option?**

    A. Aspirin, nitroglycerin, morphine, and analgesia
    B. IV heparin and thrombolytic
    C. CT angiogram of the abdomen
    D. Percutaneous coronary intervention

8. **A 78-year-old male patient presents to ER in hemorrhagic shock. Initial assessment revealed the cause of shock is ruptured abdominal aortic aneurysm. What is the most crucial approach?**

    A. Endovascular aortic repair
    B. Insertion of resuscitative endovascular balloon occlusion of aorta (REBOA)
    C. Open retroperitoneal approach and
    D. Open midline approach and supraceliac aortic cross-clamp

9. **A 66-year-old female patient is taken to the OR urgently to repair a symptomatic 9-cm abdominal aortic aneurysm (AAA). During abdominal exploration, acute calculous cholecystitis was found. What would be the most appropriate decision in dealing with this finding?**

    A. Cholecystectomy then retroperitoneal AAA repair

    B. AAA repair and perform percutaneous cholecystostomy tube immediately postoperatively

    C. AAA repair then cholecystectomy after complete graft coverage

    D. Retroperitoneal AAA repair and then cholecystectomy to avoid contamination of the graft

10. **A 52-year-old female patient with chronic burn nonhealing wound over both legs presented to the clinic with an ulcer over the medial malleolus of her left ankle. Her ankle-brachial index (ABI) is 1.05. What is the most likely type of ulcer?**

    A. Malignant

    B. Traumatic

    C. Neuropathic

    D. Venous

11. **A 63-year-old male patient is admitted to the emergency department five days after a laparoscopic Heller myotomy for achalasia with fever, chills, and epigastric and left shoulder pain. His temperature is 39°C, white blood cell count is 22,000, and hemoglobin is 15 g/dL. A CT scan shows a left subphrenic fluid collection and left lower lobe consolidation. What is the cause of the clinical scenario?**

   A. Left lower lobe aspiration pneumonia

   B. Distal esophageal perforation

   C. Ischemia of the gastric fundus due to short gastric ligation

   D. Infected splenic hematoma from splenic capsule injury

12. **A 54-year-old male patient presents with progressive dysphagia and regurgitation of undigested food. Barium swallow showed dilated esophagus with gradual distal narrowing of the esophagus. What is the most likely diagnosis?**

   A. Chronic fungal esophagitis

   B. Diffuse esophageal spasm

   C. Esophageal web

   D. Achalasia

13. **A 55-year-old female patient with a long history of a gastro-esophageal reflux disease had an endoscopic examination and biopsy of the lower esophagus. The histology report showed evidence of intestinal metaplasia. Which type of esophageal cancer would be prevents with appropriate treatment?**

   A. Squamous cell carcinoma
   B. Non-Hodgkin's lymphoma
   C. Gastrointestinal stromal tumor (GIST)
   D. Adenocarcinoma

14. **A 41-year-old male patient complains of regurgitation of saliva and undigested food. Barium swallow reveals a "bird's beak" deformity. What would be the best diagnostic test?**

   A. Upper GI endoscopy and multiple biopsies
   B. Manometry
   C. CT chest with oral contrast
   D. pH study of the stomach

15. **A 25-year-old healthy female patient presents to the clinic with right hand pain and numbness especially in cold weather. CT chest and neck revealed first rib compressing the right subclavian artery. What is the best treatment option?**

   A. Conservative therapy with analgesia, physiotherapy, and work tasks modification
   B. Heparinization and limb rest with elevation
   C. Angiogram and stenting of the subclavian artery
   D. Decompressive surgery

Answer Key: 1 – B, 2 – A, 3 – C, 4 – D, 5 – A, 6 – C, 7 – C, 8 – D, 9 – C, 10 – A, 11 – B, 12 – D, 13 – D, 14 – B, 15 – D

ABOUT THE AUTHOR

Hassan Bukhari is a general and trauma surgeon and an intensivist. Dr. Bukhari is an associate professor at Umm Al-Qura University, Saudi Arabia. He enjoys discovering different methods in teaching medical knowledge and skills and loves writing multiple-choice questions (MCQs). Dr. Bukhari is passionate about understanding how MCQs are constructed and solved. Dr. Bukhari went through thousands of MCQs and experienced a lot of MCQ examinations during his medical school, residency, and fellowship, and licensing exams. When he came back to his home university, he became responsible for constructing and supervising many MCQ exam for different under – and postgraduate years. Dr. Bukhari decided to write this book to help under – and postgraduates understand how to tackle MCQ exams and improve their scores. His experience in writing books is remarkable after he published his well-known book in general surgery called "Puzzles in General Surgery" first and second editions.